ALL SORTS O
HEALTHY DISHES
THE MEDITERRANEAN WAY

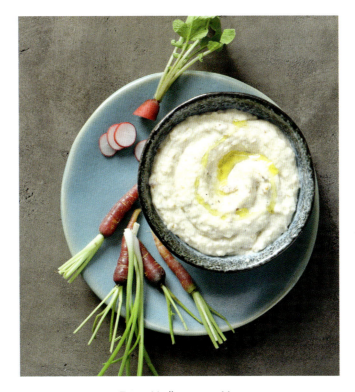

To my Mediterranean Man
Thanks for all the special memories that helped inspire this book.
Here's to staying healthy.

CHANTAL LASCARIS

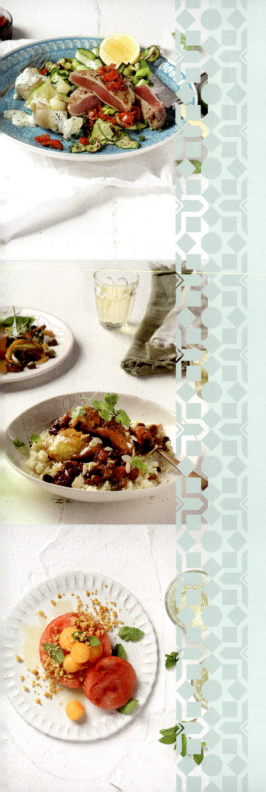

Published in 2017 by Struik Lifestyle
an imprint of Penguin Random House South Africa (Pty) Ltd
Company Reg. No. 1953/000441/07
The Estuaries, 4 Oxbow Crescent, Century Avenue, Century City, 7441
PO Box 1144, Cape Town 8000, South Africa

www.penguinrandomhouse.co.za

ISBN 978-1-43230-823-0

Publisher: Linda de Villiers
Managing editor: Cecilia Barfield
Design manager and designer: Beverley Dodd
Proofreader and indexer: Joy Clack
Photographer: Henk Hattingh
Photographer's assistants: Jomeri Mouton
Stylist: Luisa Farelo
Stylist's assistant: Zani Malan

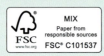

FSC
MIX
Paper from
responsible sources
FSC® C101537

Reproduction by Hirt & Carter Cape (Pty) Ltd
Printed and bound in China by RR Donnelley Asia Printing Solutions, Ltd.

CONTENTS

INTRODUCTION

I've been on many diets with varying degrees of success – great success for the diet's promoter, less success for me.

You can get a lot out of a diet, including all the things you can do without, such as added cholesterol, additional rolls around the waist, shaky hands and sweaty palms. What you really want are healthy meals that leave you feeling good. Which brings me to the Mediterranean and its sunshine cuisine.

I am lucky enough to have travelled regularly to various Mediterranean countries. Every time I returned home I felt healthier than before I left, which led me to conduct my own research into the Mediterranean way of eating. I wanted to find a way to incorporate elements of this culinary approach into my own quest for a healthy lifestyle once back in South Africa.

It was surprisingly easy. After all, much of South Africa – and the Cape most particularly – has a similar climate to many of the countries along the Mediterranean Sea and produces many of the ingredients that are integral to this way of eating.

But before I go any further, I should explain that the Mediterranean diet is not a diet at all; at least, not in the calorie-counting sense of the word. Rather, it is a way of eating and a lifestyle. Nor is it fancy food; originally it was considered peasant food, so it's good and wholesome and the cooking techniques are simple. Ingredients that make up a typical Mediterranean meal are close to nature and seasonal, so they're enjoyed at their tastiest and healthiest.

In the past, eating seasonally was the only way people could eat. Nowadays, it's the only way we should eat, for our own good and the good of the planet.

There is a worldwide trend towards Mediterranean cuisine and lifestyle. Countless studies have shown that a traditional Mediterranean diet can help reduce the chances of developing type 2 diabetes and high blood pressure, while bringing down elevated levels of cholesterol – all chronic health problems in South Africa. Sunshine cuisine includes plenty of vegetables, fruits, beans, brown rice, white meat and fish. There is also a strong emphasis on good fats such as olive oil and nuts. All these products are readily available in South Africa, or we have ingredients that can easily be substituted.

Happily, it's also an affordable way of eating. In many Mediterranean dishes beans or lentils are the main source of protein and serving plants and whole grains is less expensive than serving packaged or processed foods.

THE PRINCIPLES OF A MEDITERRANEAN CULINARY LIFESTYLE

Eat fruits and vegetables as well as whole grains, nuts and legumes

A large part of every meal should consist of fruits and vegetables. Soups, crudités and salads can all amp up your plant-based intake. You can continue to 'freshen up' by adding vegetables to other dishes. While you're at it, switch to wholegrain bread, pasta and rice. Nuts and fruit are perfect snacks.

Replace butter with olive oil

Olive oil is a 'healthy fat' as it provides monounsaturated fat, which can help to reduce LDL cholesterol levels. It also contains phenols (strong antioxidants that fight free radicals and reduce inflammation). Use olive oil for dipping instead of sodium-rich processed dips and sauces. It should be the predominant fat in your diet.

Use herbs and spices to flavour food

Salt is a very unhealthy way of flavouring food. It's high in sodium and promotes high blood pressure. Rather switch to herbs, spices and garlic to add a delicious taste to your dishes. Herbs also have many health benefits – another reason to use them instead of merely adding salt.

Limit red meat

For most people in South Africa this is probably the most daunting aspect of Mediterranean eating as we are accustomed to consuming large amounts of red meat. In contrast, Mediterranean peoples traditionally had limited access to this source of dietary protein due to the difficulty in rearing large herds of cattle in their rugged terrain. A cow eats 10—15kg of grass a day. Fodder like that was simply not available. Lambs, sheep and goats were reared instead. For improved health we need to limit our intake of red meat to once or twice a week, also ensuring that it's as lean as possible.

Eat fish and poultry

Fish is a major source of omega-3 fatty acids and is rich in other nutrients such as vitamin D and selenium. Fish and poultry are high in protein and low in saturated fat.

Drink red wine (optional)

A glass of wine a day can aid digestion (but remember, moderation is key). Red wine contains antioxidants as well as anti-inflammatory compounds and can help prevent heart disease.

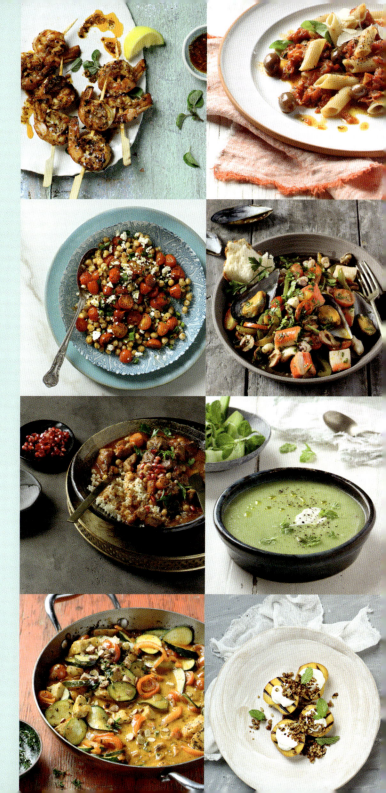

Exercise regularly

People along the Mediterranean exercise naturally, as part of their everyday lives. There's nothing like working the land for keeping fit. So we need to incorporate regular exercise into our modern lifestyles. It involves more than just hitting the gym for one hour three times a week. The easiest way to support the fitness habit is to walk more. Try parking your car further away from the shopping centre entrance. Take the stairs instead of the lift. Remember, to keep your weight down you must burn off more calories than you consume.

Share meals with others

One of the essential ingredients of this lifestyle is the custom of sharing meals with others. No sitting in front of the TV, quickly consuming a microwaved premade meal for Mediterranean families. They sit down together for a leisurely meal. Mealtimes are perfect for family bonding and reducing stress, a factor that contributes to many health conditions and detracts from quality of life.

SO YOU THINK YOU DON'T HAVE TIME FOR THIS?

By now you're probably thinking, 'This is all very well, but how on earth can I follow this lifestyle when I don't have time to make my own meals?' Relax! The dishes I've formulated are based on a number of classic ideas from France, Greece, Italy, Morocco, Spain and Turkey. They all contain readily available ingredients while the recipes are easy to follow.

To make your life even easier, I've suggested the vegetables and side dishes you might like to serve with each main course, to ensure that you will get enough of the plant-based foodstuffs that make this such a healthy way of eating.

More than 20 countries border the Mediterranean Sea, but I take my inspiration from France, Greece, Italy, Morocco, Spain and Turkey. This allows for plenty of variety, but keeps things manageable.

I have to admit that fluffy soufflés, sauce-rich lasagna, salami-topped pizzas with extra cheese and long white loaves of bread slathered with butter all originate from Mediterranean lands as well, but they certainly don't form part of the traditional Mediterranean diet, so forget about them.

South Africa has the climate, the foods and ingredients. So sit back, inwardly digest and enjoy.

Bon Appetit!

Chantal Lascaris

CHANTAL LASCARIS

GENERAL CONVERSIONS

METRIC TO CUPS/SPOONS

Metric	Teaspoons	Metric	Cups
2ml	¼ tsp	60ml	¼ cup
3ml	½ tsp	80ml	⅓ cup
5ml	1 tsp	125ml	½ cup
10ml	2 tsp	160ml	⅔ cup
20ml	4 tsp	200ml	¾ cup
		250ml	1 cup
Metric	Tablespoons	375ml	1½ cups
15ml	1 Tbsp	500ml	2 cups
30ml	2 Tbsp	750ml	3 cups
45ml	3 Tbsp	1 litre	4 cups
60ml	4 Tbsp		

SERVINGS

Please note that all recipes serve 4 people.

BRINJALS: TO DÉGORGE OR NOT TO DÉGORGE

Traditionally, brinjals (also known as aubergines or eggplants) needed to be dégorged – the process of salting them to draw out the bitter liquid. Large (often older) brinjals contain brown seeds, which are the source of the bitter liquid. However, some of the newer varieties of brinjal or smaller fruits have few seeds and do not need to be dégorged. If you're unsure and would prefer to do so, slice the brinjal and season it generously with salt. Leave the the slices until beads of moisture form on the surface. Rinse the slices thoroughly and pat them dry.

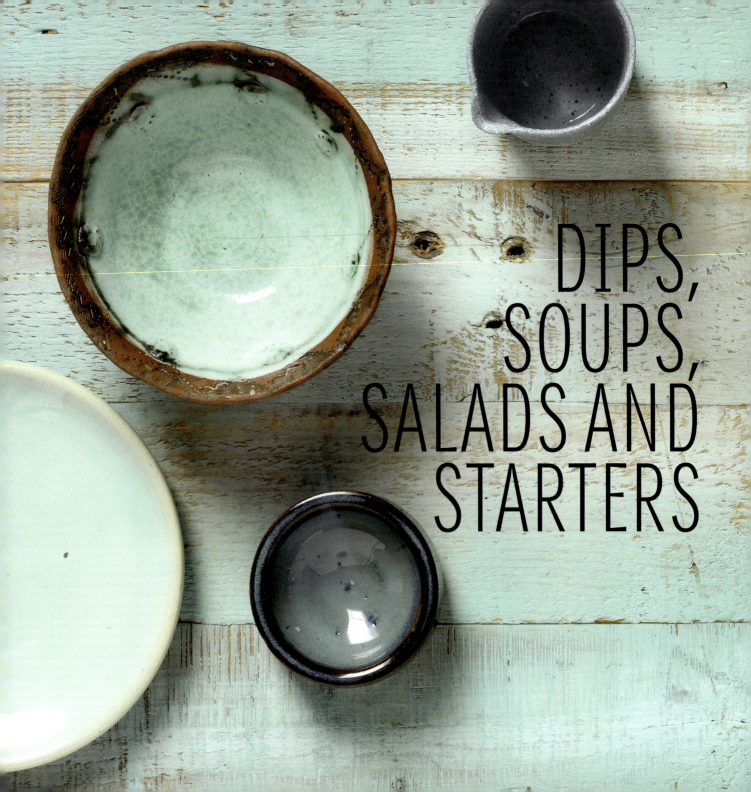

DIPS, SOUPS, SALADS AND STARTERS

Each Mediterranean country has its own name for it, but one thing they all have in common is their love of the convivial habit of getting together to eat small portions, either as a precursor to the meal, or at a table heaving under the weight of multiple small dishes. Traditionally, a small plate of food was served with an apéritif, such as raki, ouzo or wine.

For the first course, I prefer to keep the dishes simple, light and fresh so as not to spoil the appetite for what's still to come. Dishes suggested here are interchangeable, may be hot or cold, but all are healthy and, above all, delicious. Some of the simplest are also the most successful. Many can be served on individual plates or as part of platters. No matter how the dishes are presented, this course creates an instant, relaxed atmosphere. So why not try a watermelon and beetroot gazpacho on a hot, sun-drenched day or, for an elegant dinner, up the tempo with artichoke and tomato towers? No matter what dish you choose, these sun-soaked recipes are colourful and nutritious.

DID YOU KNOW?
- 'Antipasto' means 'before the meal' in Italian.
- In France, 'hors d'oeuvre' has a similar meaning.
- In Spain, the word 'tapa' means 'cover' or 'coaster', a reference to the tradition of covering the wine with a small plate of food. This was made law in the 1200s when King Alfonso banned the tavernas from serving alcohol without food. A cover also had the practical benefit of stopping fruit flies from settling in the wine.
- Meze is frequently found in the cuisine of countries from the former Ottoman Empire (including Greece, Turkey *et al*) and comes from the word 'meze', which means 'taste' or 'snack'.

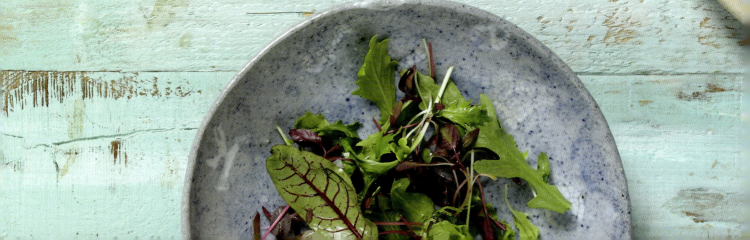

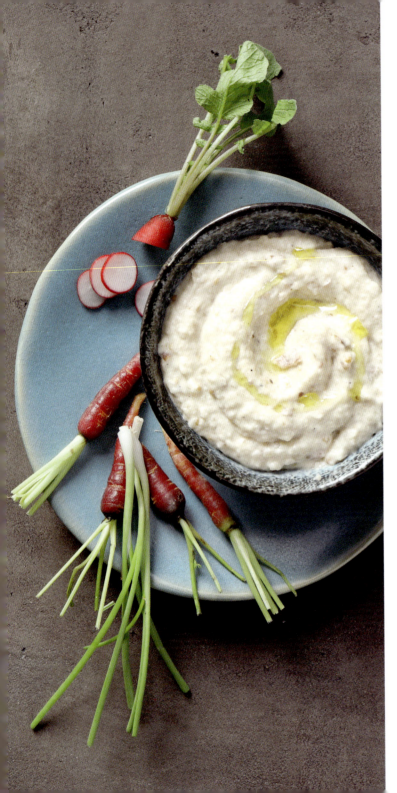

BRINJAL DIP

CREAMY, GARLICKY AND YUMMY IS THE BEST WAY TO DESCRIBE THIS DIP. BRINJALS (ALSO KNOWN AS AUBERGINES OR EGGPLANTS) ARE SYNONYMOUS WITH THE MEDITERRANEAN AND TRADITIONALLY THIS DIP WOULD HAVE A SMOKY FLAVOUR. THIS IS A CHEAT'S VERSION THAT TASTES AS HEAVENLY AS THE MORE TRADITIONAL BABA GANOUSH. IT WILL KEEP IN THE FRIDGE FOR A FEW DAYS. USE HALF MAYONNAISE AND HALF YOGHURT TO CUT BACK ON SOME OF THE CALORIES.

1 unpeeled brinjal, chopped
1 onion, chopped
olive oil for sautéing and drizzling
1 tsp crushed garlic
2 Tbsp mayonnaise
1 Tbsp double thick Greek (or plain) yoghurt
juice of ½ lemon
salt and pepper to taste

1. Gently sauté the brinjal and onion in a little oil until soft.
2. Remove from the heat and allow to cool.
3. Using a hand-held blender, mash the mixture with the garlic.
4. Stir in the mayonnaise and yoghurt until well mixed.
5. Add the lemon juice, salt and pepper and stir through.
6. Taste, then add extra lemon juice or mayonnaise if you'd like more tang.
7. Drizzle with olive oil.

RED PEPPER & CASHEW DIP

THIS IS SO TASTY YOU'LL WANT TO SMEAR IT ON MORE THAN JUST CRACKERS. BELL PEPPERS ORIGINALLY DERIVED THEIR NAME FROM SPANISH EXPLORERS WHO WERE SEARCHING FOR PEPPERCORN PLANTS TO PRODUCE BLACK PEPPER. BUT RED PEPPERS DON'T HAVE THE HEAT OF PEPPERCORNS AS THEY DON'T CONTAIN CAPSAICIN, WHICH IS WHAT MAKES PEPPER HOT. RED PEPPERS ARE ACTUALLY THE SWEETEST OF THE THREE BELL PEPPERS.

3 red peppers
½ cup roasted cashew nuts
2 tsp minced garlic
½ cup olive oil
½ tsp dried thyme
1 Tbsp lemon juice
salt and pepper to taste

1. Preheat the oven to 180°C.
2. Slice the peppers in half, remove the seeds and membranes and place on a baking tray, skin-side up. Bake in the oven for about 20 minutes.
3. Remove and allow to cool before removing the skins.
4. In a blender, first blitz the cashew nuts then add the remaining ingredients and blend until smooth.
5. Check the seasoning, then garnish as desired. Store in the refrigerator.

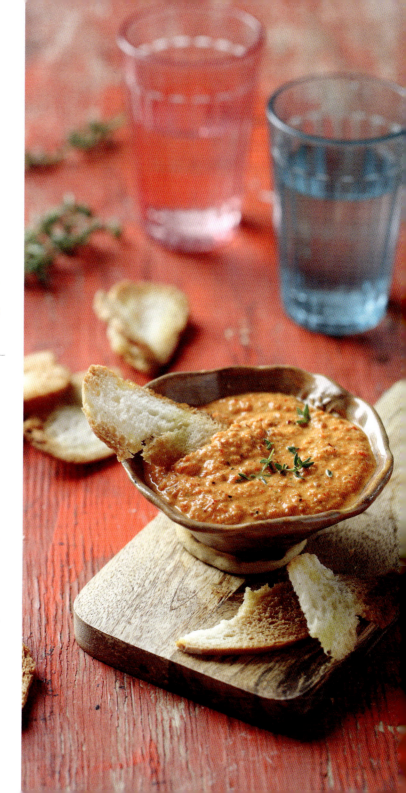

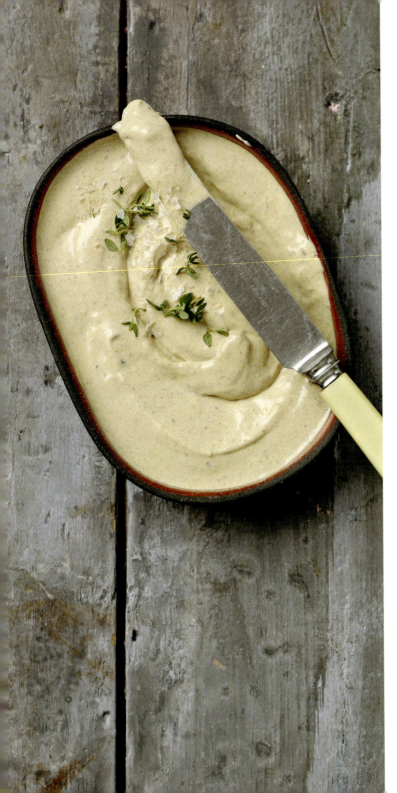

OYSTER PÂTÉ

NOT ONLY ARE OYSTERS NUTRITIONALLY WELL BALANCED, CONTAINING PROTEIN, CARBOHYDRATES AND LIPIDS, THEY ARE ALSO A GOOD SOURCE OF VITAMINS A, B1, B2, B3, C AND D. AS JONATHAN SWIFT IS OFTEN CREDITED AS SAYING, 'HE WAS A BOLD MAN THAT FIRST ATE AN OYSTER.'

1 x 85g can smoked oysters
1 Tbsp tangy mayonnaise
Tabasco sauce to taste (±10 drops)
2 Tbsp good quality tomato sauce
½ cup cream cheese
salt and pepper to taste
fresh herbs for garnishing

1. Using a hand-held blender, blitz together all the ingredients, except the salt and pepper.
2. Season lightly.
3. Transfer the pâté to a ramekin and garnish with fresh herbs.

PETITS POIS PÂTÉ

THE PETIT POIS IS A YOUNG, DE-HULLED PEA. IT WAS PART OF A COMPOSITION THAT PABLO PICASSO PAINTED IN 1911, KNOWN AS 'LE PIGEON AUX PETITS POIS'. IT WAS STOLEN FROM A FRENCH MUSEUM IN 2010 AND REMAINS MISSING. WHAT'S NOT MISSING HERE, HOWEVER, IS THE POWERHOUSE OF FLAVOUR AND GOODNESS THAT THIS LITTLE PÂTÉ PROVIDES.

3 eggs
3 Tbsp olive oil
1½ medium onions, chopped
½ cup roughly chopped green beans
1 cup frozen petits pois
¾ cup halved walnuts
salt and pepper to taste

1. Boil the eggs for 5 minutes, then leave them to cool before peeling and cutting into quarters.
2. In a saucepan, heat the oil, add the onions and fry gently until softened.
3. Stir in the green beans and petits pois.
4. Continue to cook until the beans are soft.
5. Place the walnuts and eggs in a blender or food processor, then blend until they form a paste. Add the onion, bean and pea mixture then pulse to form a coarse pâté.
6. Season with salt and pepper.
7. To serve, place a spoonful of the pâté onto slices of Melba toast or crackers of your choice.

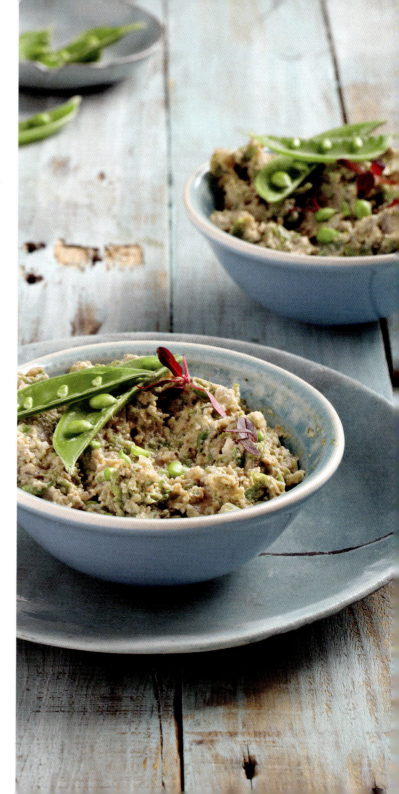

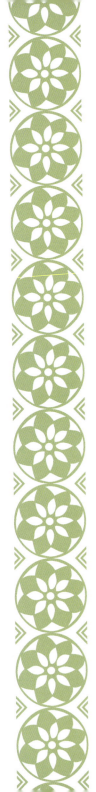

WATERMELON & BEETROOT GAZPACHO

ORIGINATING IN THE ANDALUSIAN REGION OF SPAIN, GAZPACHO HAS BEEN REFERRED TO AS A LIQUID SALAD. IT'S PARTICULARLY ENJOYABLE DURING THE HOT SUMMER MONTHS. THIS UNUSUAL COMBINATION TASTES AS COOL AND DELICIOUS AS IT SOUNDS.

1 beetroot

350g watermelon flesh, seeds removed

½ cup chopped, peeled cucumber

1 spring onion

½ x 400g can chopped tomatoes

1 tomato, chopped

1 cup water

1 clove garlic

salt and pepper to taste

plain yoghurt for serving

fresh mint leaves for garnishing

1. Boil the beetroot in water until soft, then leave to cool. Peel and chop.
2. Combine all the ingredients, except the seasoning, in a blender or food processor and blend to a purée.
3. Season with salt and pepper.
4. Leave to chill in the fridge.
5. When ready to serve, spoon a dollop of yoghurt over each serving and garnish with a few mint leaves.

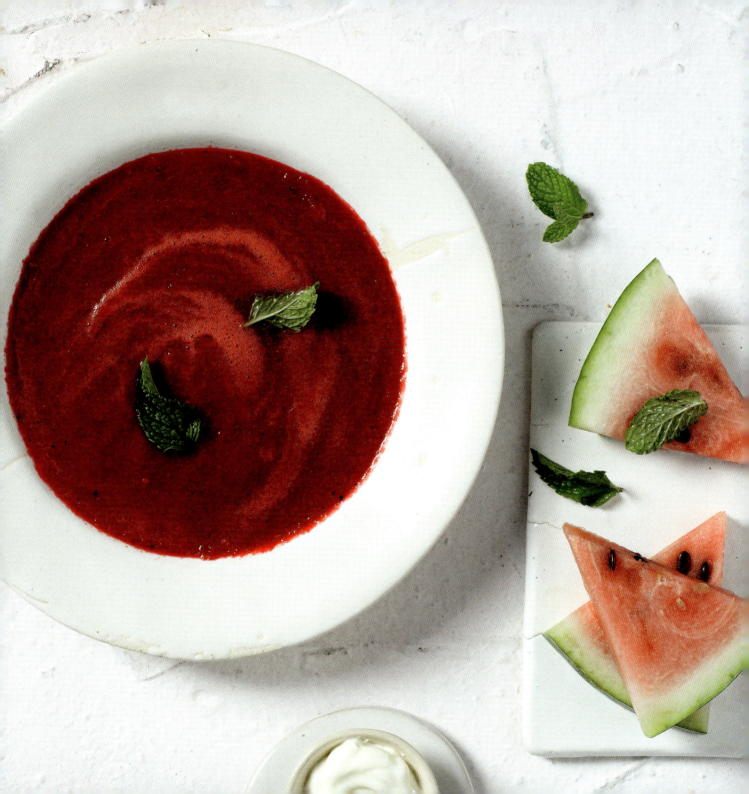

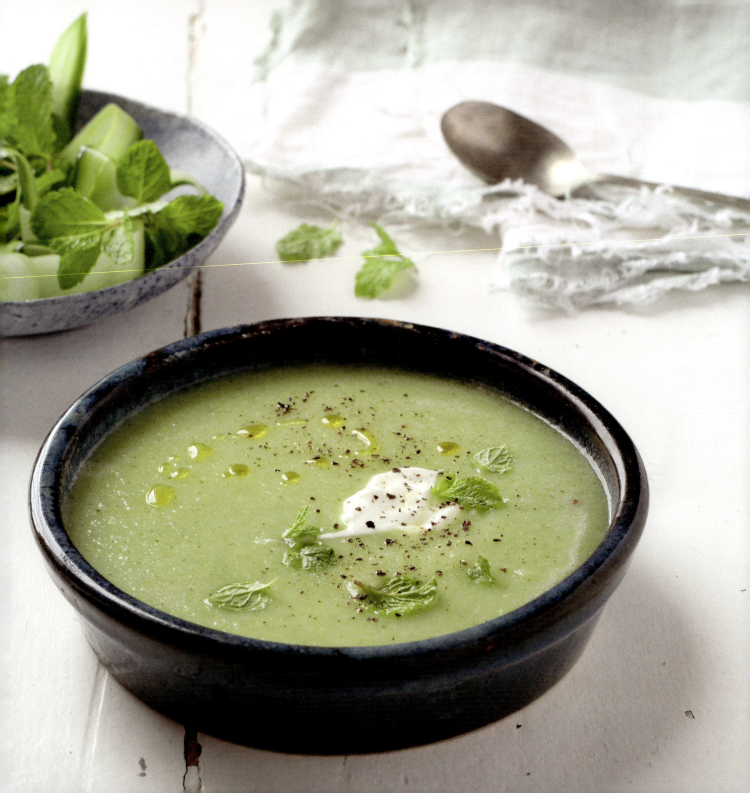

CHILLED CUCUMBER SOUP

IN ROMAN TIMES CUCUMBERS WERE GROWN IN GREENHOUSES FOR EMPEROR TIBERIUS TO ENJOY ALL YEAR ROUND. IT WAS ONLY IN THE 1800S THAT THE VARIETIES OF CUCUMBER WE ENJOY TODAY BEGAN TO BE HYBRIDIZED. WHAT BETTER WAY TO ENJOY OUR SUNSHINE THAN WITH A BOWL OF CHILLED CUCUMBER SOUP, WHICH COOLS THE BLOOD AS WELL AS THE PALATE.

---

1 cucumber, peeled and chopped
1 baby potato, boiled
¼ cup chicken stock
1 Tbsp finely chopped fresh mint
salt and pepper to taste
plain yoghurt for serving
fresh herbs for garnishing
olive oil for drizzling

1. Using a blender, blitz all the ingredients, except the seasoning, together.
2. Season with salt and pepper.
3. Leave to chill in the fridge for at least an hour before serving.
4. Add a dollop of yoghurt to each portion, garnish with fresh herbs and drizzle with olive oil.

ARTICHOKE SOUP

THE DELICATE FLAVOURS OF ARTICHOKE ARE PERFECTLY PAIRED WITH POTATOES TO CREATE A SMOOTH, SILKY SOUP. NO FLAVOUR IS SACRIFICED BY THE OMISSION OF CREAM BECAUSE GREEK YOGHURT WILL PROVIDE THE RICHNESS WITHOUT THE CALORIES. SITTING AROUND A WARM FIRE WHILE TUCKING INTO A COMFORTING BOWL OF SOUP … NOTHING COULD BE BETTER. DON'T WORRY ABOUT WASTING ANY LEFTOVER PARMESAN CRUMBLE; KEEP IT REFRIGERATED IN AN AIRTIGHT CONTAINER.

---

1 onion, chopped

1 Tbsp olive oil

1 x 410g can artichoke hearts or bottoms in brine

2 cups chicken stock

1 medium unpeeled potato, chopped

2–3 tsp cornflour, mixed with a little water

1 cup milk

salt and pepper to taste

Greek yoghurt for serving

chopped fresh herbs for garnishing

PARMESAN CRUMBLE (OPTIONAL)

1½ Tbsp grated Parmesan

1 Tbsp butter

3 Tbsp cake flour

salt and pepper to taste

¼ tsp dried thyme

1. If using, first prepare the Parmesan crumble. Use your fingers to rub together the Parmesan, butter and flour until the mixture resembles breadcrumbs.
2. Season with salt and pepper and mix in the thyme.
3. Spread the mixture on a non-stick baking tray and place under the grill for about 3 minutes, stirring once, until it is golden and crispy.
4. In a saucepan, gently fry the onion in the olive oil until softened.
5. Halve the artichokes and reserve the brine.
6. Add the chicken stock, 1 cup of the reserved artichoke brine, the artichoke halves and the chopped potato to the saucepan. Bring to the boil and simmer for about 7 minutes, making sure the potato is cooked through.
7. Remove from the heat and leave to cool slightly.
8. Purée the mixture, then gradually stir in the cornflour and milk until well blended.
9. Simmer for another few minutes and season to taste.
10. To serve, add a dollop of Greek yoghurt to each bowl, sprinkle over some Parmesan crumble (if using) and chopped fresh herbs. Serve immediately.

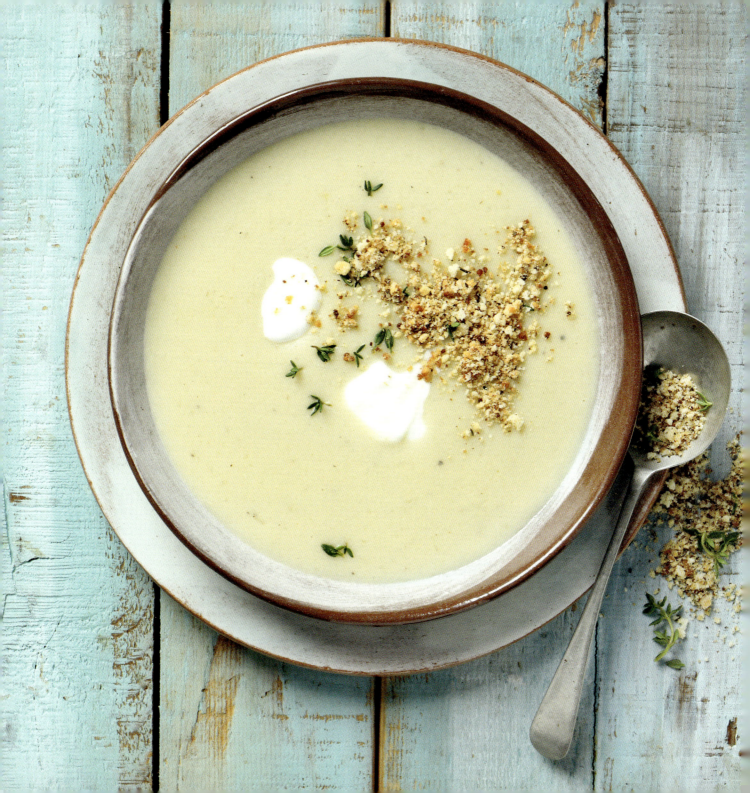

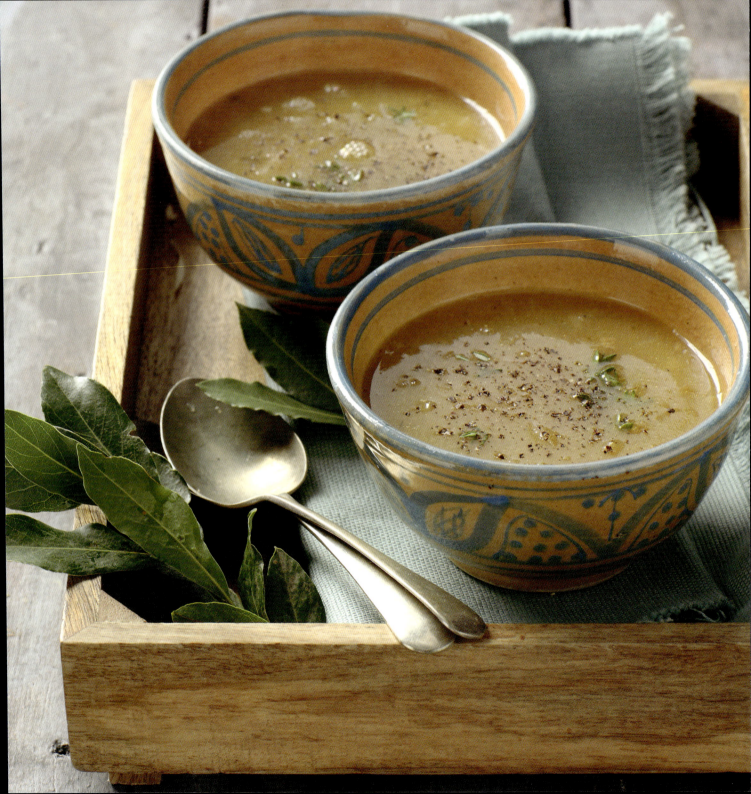

FRENCH ONION SOUP

CARAMELISED ONIONS THAT TURN GOLDEN AND MELLOW ARE THE KEY TO A GOOD FRENCH ONION SOUP, WHICH ORIGINATED IN ITS CURRENT FORM IN THE 18TH CENTURY. THIS IS A HEARTY, WARMING SOUP THAT IS PERFECT TO SERVE TO GUESTS. FOR A MORE INDULGENT OPTION, SERVE WITH PARMESAN SHAVINGS OR GRILLED PARMESAN CROUTONS ON TOP.

2 Tbsp olive oil
2–3 large onions, finely sliced
1 Tbsp cake flour
1½ cups water
¼ cup dry white wine
2 cups chicken stock
2 dried bay leaves
1 tsp dried thyme
salt and pepper to taste
Parmesan shavings for serving (optional)

GRILLED PARMESAN CROUTONS (OPTIONAL)
½ cup grated Parmesan
4 slices French bread

1. Add the oil and onions to a saucepan and cook for about 20 minutes, stirring often until the onions are soft and almost caramelised.
2. Mix in the flour. Add the water, wine, stock, bay leaves and thyme, and bring to the boil.
3. Leave to simmer for approximately 20 minutes.
4. Using a slotted spoon, remove half of the onions from the saucepan. Blitz them to a purée with a blender, then stir back into the soup. Simmer for another 5 minutes.
5. Season with salt and pepper and remove the bay leaves.
6. Serve decorated with Parmesan shavings or grilled Parmesan croutons (if using).
7. To make the croutons, sprinkle the Parmesan onto each slice of bread.
8. Place under the grill until the cheese starts to melt. Remove and serve.

ITALIAN *PICCOLO* SALAD

'*PICCOLO*' MEANS 'SMALL' OR 'LITTLE', WHICH APTLY DESCRIBES THE COLOURFUL BABY CARROTS THAT ARE THE STAR INGREDIENT OF THIS SALAD. THEY'RE COMPLEMENTED BY THE MIX OF COLOURFUL LEAVES AND SALTY PARMESAN. A DRESSING OF MUSTARD AND HONEY, FLAVOURED WITH CLASSIC ITALIAN ORIGANUM, ROUNDS OFF THIS LITTLE DISH WITH BIG FLAVOURS.

1 Tbsp olive oil
200g rainbow baby carrots
1 cup mixed salad leaves
50g spring onions, chopped
1 Tbsp roughly chopped fresh basil
1 Tbsp roughly chopped fresh parsley
¼ cup Parmesan shavings

DRESSING
¼ tsp prepared Dijon mustard
1 Tbsp white wine vinegar
3 Tbsp olive oil
¼ tsp dried origanum
½ tsp honey
¼ tsp crushed garlic
salt and pepper to taste

1. Heat the olive oil in a griddle pan and grill the carrots until slightly charred but not too soft. Remove and set aside to cool.
2. In a salad bowl, mix together the salad leaves, spring onions, basil and parsley.
3. Arrange the carrots over the leaves.
4. Blend the dressing ingredients together and pour over, making sure the salad is well coated.
5. Scatter the Parmesan shavings over the salad.
6. Serve chilled.

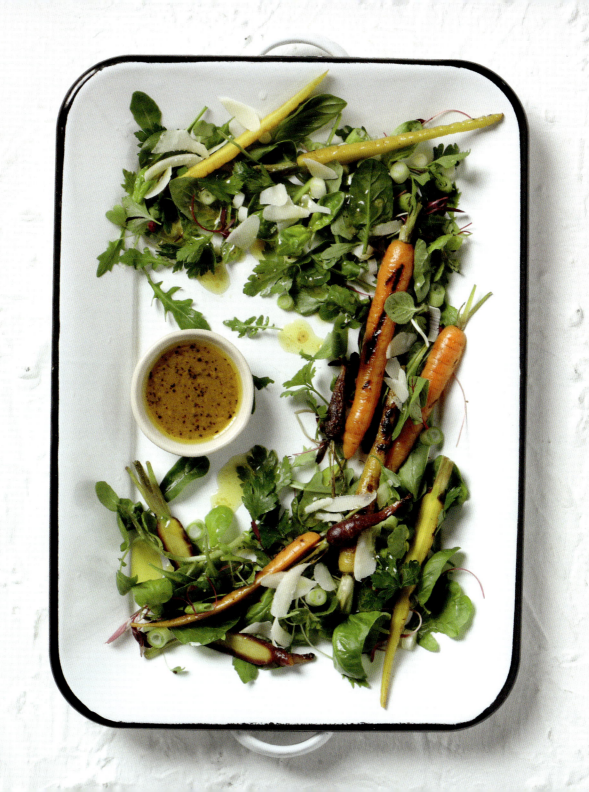

BULGUR WHEAT SALAD

BULGUR WHEAT WILL PROVIDE YOU WITH A GOOD DOSE OF YOUR DIETARY FIBRE NEEDS AND IS ALSO LOW IN FAT. IT'S USED EXTENSIVELY IN MIDDLE EASTERN DISHES AND IS PERFECT AS THE BASE FOR A HEALTHY, FILLING SALAD. THE APRICOTS ADD SOME SWEETNESS BUT THE MINT ALSO HAS A STARRING ROLE.

½ onion, finely chopped
½ tsp minced garlic
olive oil
1½ cups water
½ cup bulgur wheat
⅓ cup chopped dried apricots
¼ cup chopped pistachios
1 cup fresh rocket leaves
¼ cup chopped fresh coriander
¼ cup chopped fresh mint
½ Tbsp grated lemon zest

DRESSING
1 Tbsp lemon juice
3 Tbsp olive oil
a small pinch of sugar
salt and pepper to taste

1. In a frying pan, gently sauté the onion and garlic in a little olive oil until softened.
2. Place the water, bulgur wheat and apricots in a saucepan and simmer for about 20 minutes or until the water has been completely absorbed. Remove and place in a salad bowl.
3. Add the onion and garlic, rocket, coriander and mint and mix through.
4. Whisk the dressing ingredients together and pour over the salad, coating well.
5. Refrigerate until ready to serve.
6. Just before serving, sprinkle over the lemon zest.

TOMATO & FENNEL SALAD

FENNEL WAS GROWN BY THE ANCIENT ROMANS, WHO TREASURED IT FOR ITS AROMATIC FRUITS AND EDIBLE SHOOTS. IT IS ALSO ONE OF THE PRIMARY INGREDIENTS OF ABSINTHE, A POWERFUL ALCOHOLIC DRINK. NO HALLUCINATING HERE WHERE THE FENNEL'S STRONG ANISE FLAVOUR IS COUNTERBALANCED WITH THE MINT AND PARSLEY.

2 fennel bulbs, sliced
1 cup halved mixed small tomatoes
2 tsp chopped fresh mint
1 tsp chopped fresh parsley
2 Tbsp chopped baby spinach leaves
1 tsp slivered almonds, roasted

DRESSING
3 Tbsp olive oil
2 tsp white wine vinegar
¼ tsp honey
salt and pepper to taste

1. Place the fennel in a salad bowl with the tomatoes, mint, parsley and spinach leaves. Toss well.
2. Whisk the dressing ingredients together and pour over the salad, coating well.
3. Refrigerate until ready to serve.
4. Just before serving, scatter the almonds over the salad.

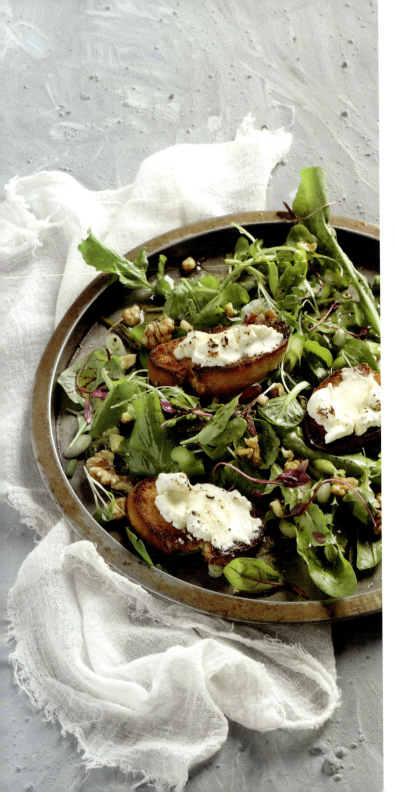

GOAT'S MILK CHEESE SALAD

GOAT'S MILK CHEESE IS A GREAT SUBSTITUTE FOR COW'S MILK CHEESE. IT IS RICHER IN VITAMINS AND MINERALS AND CONTAINS LESS LACTOSE, CALORIES, CHOLESTEROL AND FAT. WALNUTS ARE THE OLDEST KNOWN TREE FOOD, IN USE FOR SOME 12 000 YEARS. IT'S TRADITIONAL TO SERVE GOAT'S MILK CHEESE WITH WALNUTS .... SO WHY CHANGE?

8 slices goat's milk
    cheese
8 slices small baguette,
    toasted
honey
2 cups mixed salad
    greens
4 spring onions, chopped
1 Tbsp chopped walnuts

DRESSING
¼ cup olive oil
2 Tbsp white wine
    vinegar
a drizzle of honey
salt and pepper to taste

1. Place a slice of cheese onto each of the slices of baguette.
2. Add a drop of honey to each slice of cheese.
3. Place under the grill until the cheese starts to brown.
4. Mix together the salad greens, spring onions and walnuts.
5. Whisk together the dressing ingredients and pour over the salad leaves, coating well.
6. Arrange the salad leaves on a platter and place the baguette slices on top.
7. Serve immediately while the cheese is still warm.

SPINACH & RAISIN SALAD

RAISINS ARE A GREAT IN A SIDE DISH FOR ADDING FLAVOUR AND TEXTURE. THEY'RE ALSO REALLY GOOD FOR YOU BECAUSE WHEN GRAPES ARE DEHYDRATED TO PRODUCE RAISINS, THE NUTRIENTS BECOME MORE CONCENTRATED. SO A HANDFUL OF RAISINS ARE RICH IN IRON, POTASSIUM AND B VITAMINS. AS THEY'RE ALSO A GOOD SOURCE OF CARBOHYDRATES, PROVIDING ENERGY, EAT THEM IN MODERATION.

$\frac{1}{2}$ cup seedless raisins
2 Tbsp flaked almonds
2 slices white bread, crusts removed
4 Tbsp olive oil
$\frac{1}{2}$ tsp crushed garlic
2–3 cups baby spinach leaves

1. Place the raisins in a bowl and cover them with boiling water. Leave to soak for about 10 minutes.
2. Dry-roast the almonds in a pan and set aside once browned.
3. Cut the white bread into cubes.
4. Pour 2 tablespoons of the olive oil into a pan and fry the bread cubes until crispy, then set the croutons aside.
5. Drain the raisins.
6. Mix together the remaining olive oil and garlic.
7. In a salad bowl, combine the spinach leaves, raisins and almonds, then pour over the garlic oil and toss well to coat the spinach leaves.
8. Just before serving, scatter over the croutons.

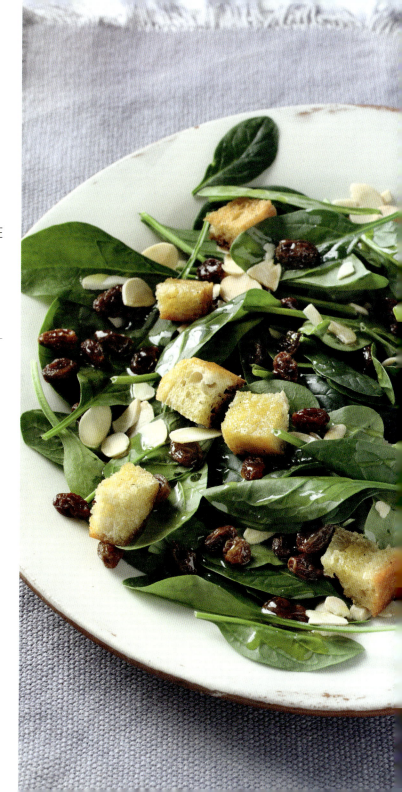

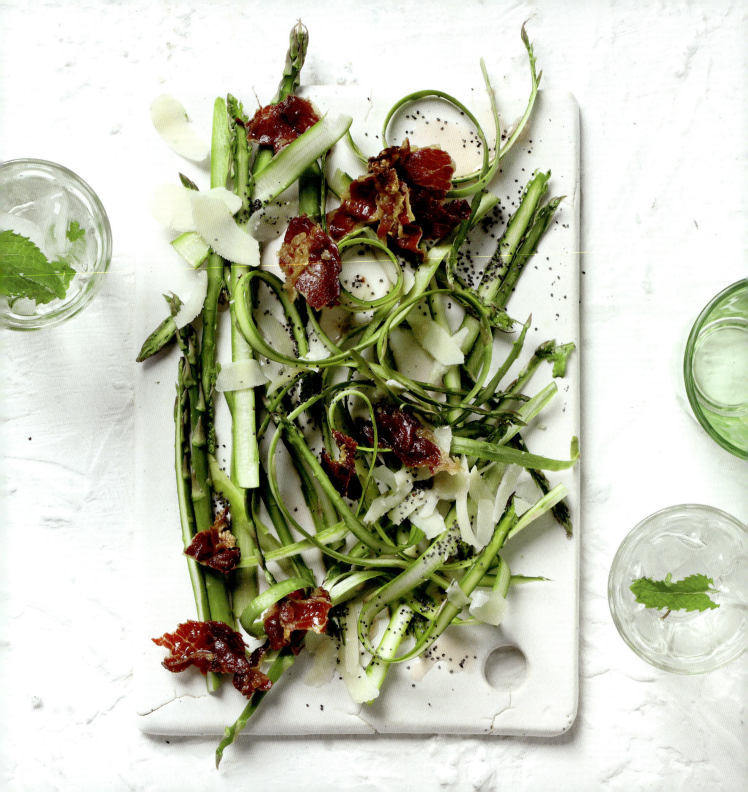

ASPARAGUS & COPPA SALAD

COPPA IS A TRADITIONAL ITALIAN PORK CUT THAT CAN BE EATEN AS IS OR COOKED. HOWEVER, ANY OTHER CURED MEAT COULD EASILY BE SUBSTITUTED. A VEGETABLE PEELER IS THE SECRET WEAPON HERE AS THE ASPARAGUS CREATES A VISUALLY APPEALING PRESENTATION THAT TASTES AS GOOD AS IT LOOKS.

6–8 large asparagus spears
juice of ½ lemon
8 slices coppa
⅓ cup Parmesan shavings
1 tsp poppy seeds for garnishing

DRESSING
¼ cup olive oil
2 Tbsp red wine vinegar
1 tsp honey
salt and pepper to taste

1. Using a vegetable peeler, finely slice the asparagus.
2. Place in a bowl and coat with the lemon juice.
3. Place the coppa on a baking tray and grill in the oven until crispy.
4. Remove and leave to cool, then break up into smaller pieces.
5. Arrange the asparagus slices on a platter and scatter over the Parmesan shavings and coppa.
6. Whisk together the dressing ingredients and pour over the salad.
7. Finally, scatter over the poppy seeds.

ARTICHOKE & TOMATO TOWERS

TECHNICALLY, AN ARTICHOKE IS A FLOWER THAT HASN'T YET BLOOMED. BUT HERE IT BLOSSOMS WHEN SERVED TOGETHER WITH TOMATOES AND MUSHROOMS. THE BALSAMIC REDUCTION PROVIDES AN ADDITIONAL FLAVOUR DIMENSION, WHILE THE ROASTED TOMATOES ADD DEPTH. BEST OF ALL, THIS DISH IS REMARKABLY EASY TO ASSEMBLE AND IS A REAL SHOW STOPPER ON THE TABLE.

2 Tbsp chopped onion
1 cup chopped button mushrooms
¼ tsp dried thyme
2 tsp olive oil
½ cup halved or quartered rosa tomatoes
¼ tsp balsamic vinegar
a pinch of sugar or a drizzle of honey

4 canned artichoke bottoms or bottled
  artichoke hearts
4 thick slices tomato
1 cup baby spinach leaves for serving
micro greens for garnishing
balsamic reduction

1. Gently fry the onion, mushrooms and thyme in a splash of the olive oil, until the onion and mushrooms have softened.
2. Add the rosa tomatoes and balsamic vinegar and sauté until the tomatoes start to soften and blister.
3. Sprinkle over the sugar or honey and stir through.
4. Remove the mixture from the pan and set aside.
5. Turn up the heat and sear the artichokes on both sides in the same pan in the remaining olive oil, then remove from the pan.
6. In the same pan, heat the tomato slices, but do not allow them to soften too much.
7. To serve, place the tomato slices on top of some spinach leaves, arrange the artichokes on top and spoon over the tomato and mushroom mixture.
8. Finally, sprinkle some micro greens on top and drizzle with balsamic reduction.

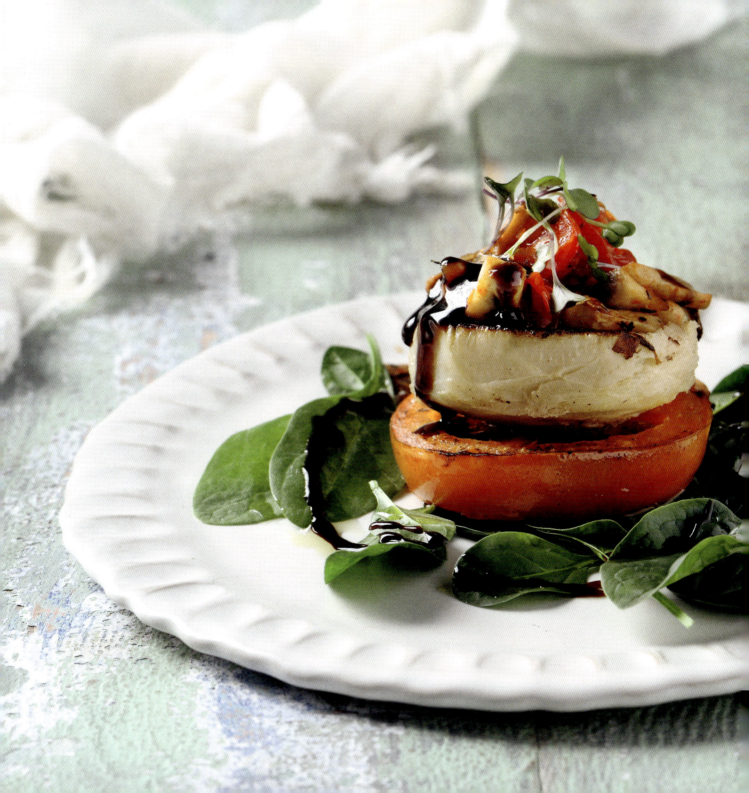

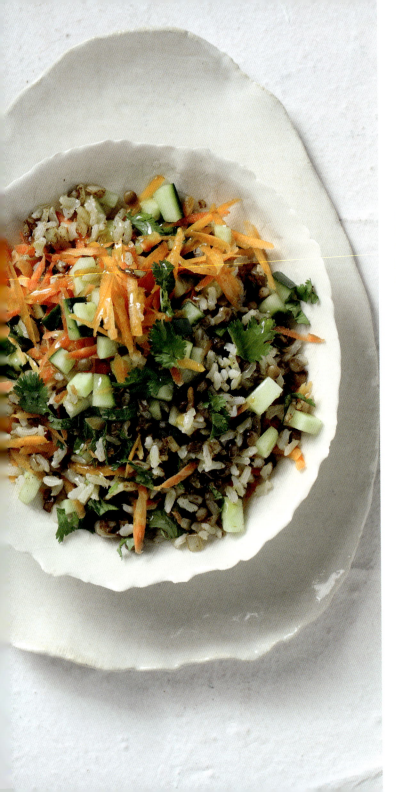

LENTIL & RICE SALAD

THIS IS A HEARTY AND HEALTHY CARBOHYDRATE SIDE DISH. THE BROWN RICE IS HIGHLY NUTRITIOUS AS IT CONTAINS PROTEINS, IS LOW IN FAT AND RICH IN MINERALS (UNLIKE WHITE RICE). THE GREEK YOGHURT IS FRAGRANTLY FLAVOURED WITH SPICES WHILE THE CORIANDER ADDS THE FINAL TOUCH.

¾ cup brown rice
2½ cups water
½ onion, finely chopped
1 tsp olive oil
½ tsp ground cinnamon
1 tsp ground cumin
1 x 410g can lentils, drained

4-cm length cucumber, diced
2 large carrots, grated
2 Tbsp Greek yoghurt
1 Tbsp chopped fresh coriander, plus extra for garnishing
salt and pepper to taste

1. In a saucepan, cover the rice with the water, bring to the boil and cook until softened. Drain and set aside.
2. Gently fry the onion in the olive oil, stir in the cinnamon and cumin and cook until the onion is translucent.
3. Combine the rice, lentils and onion mixture.
4. Add the cucumber, carrots, yoghurt and coriander, and mix well.
5. Season with salt and pepper.
6. Garnish with coriander.

MANGETOUT SALAD

HAVE YOU EVER WONDERED WHAT THE DIFFERENCE IS BETWEEN MANGETOUTS AND SUGAR SNAP PEAS? THE PEAS INSIDE A MANGETOUT DON'T SWELL, WHEREAS IN SUGAR SNAPS THEY SWELL WITHIN THE POD AND YET THE WHOLE POD REMAINS EDIBLE. BUT WHICHEVER YOU PREFER, BOTH PROVIDE A GOOD SOURCE OF FIBRE.

600g fresh mangetout
1 tsp olive oil
2 cups whole rosa
   tomatoes
100g feta cheese,
   roughly crumbled
4 Tbsp roughly chopped
   fresh parsley
1 red onion, finely sliced

¼ cup flaked almonds,
   roasted

DRESSING
¼ cup olive oil
2 Tbsp lemon juice
½ tsp honey
salt and pepper to taste

1. Place the mangetout in a pan of boiling water and simmer for about 5 minutes. Remove and refresh in cold water.
2. Heat the olive oil in a griddle pan and gently fry the tomatoes until they blister. Leave to cool.
3. Mix together the mangetout, feta, parsley, tomatoes, onion and almonds.
4. Blend the dressing ingredients together and pour over the salad, coating well. Serve chilled.

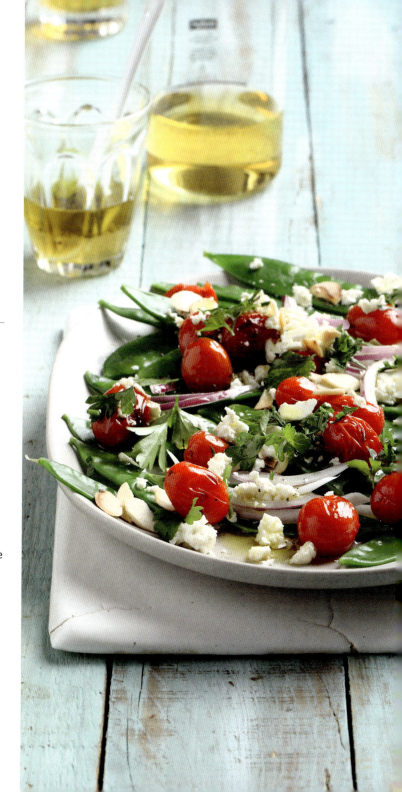

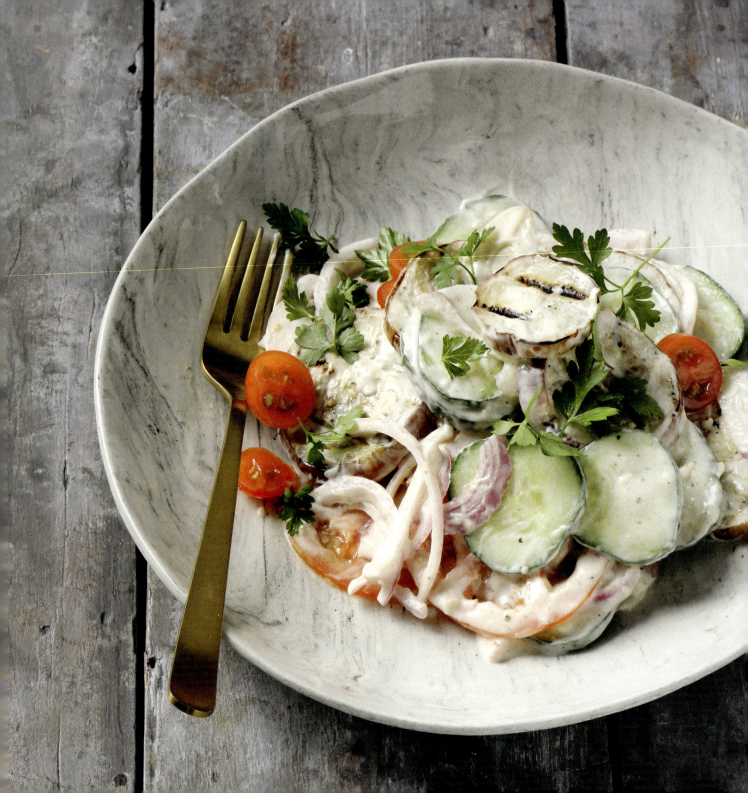

BRINJAL, TOMATO & CUCUMBER SALAD

WHAT A DELIGHT FOR THE TASTE BUDS: COOL CUCUMBER CONTRASTING WITH EARTHY BRINJAL, ALL BALANCED WITH THE SWEETNESS OF THE TOMATOES. AND THE HEALTH BENEFITS ARE THERE TOO. BRINJALS ARE RICH IN BIOFLAVONOIDS, WHICH IT'S CLAIMED MAY PREVENT STROKES. CUMIN IS A GREAT AID FOR THE DIGESTION AND IS KNOWN TO IMPROVE IMMUNITY.

¼ cup olive oil
1 medium brinjal, sliced into rounds
    ±0.5cm thick
1 large tomato, sliced
¼ cucumber, sliced
½ red onion, thinly sliced
½ tsp ground cumin

1 clove garlic, chopped
juice of ½ lemon
1 Tbsp white wine vinegar
3 Tbsp Greek yoghurt
salt and pepper to taste
sprigs of fresh parsley for garnishing

1. Brush a touch of olive oil over the brinjal slices, then grill in a preheated griddle pan, turning once.
2. Combine the tomato, cucumber, onion and brinjal slices in a bowl (if you think the tomato and brinjal slices are too large, halve them again).
3. Mix together the remaining olive oil, cumin, garlic, lemon juice, vinegar and yoghurt. Season with salt and pepper, then pour over the salad ingredients, coating well.
4. Refrigerate for at least 30 minutes before serving to allow the flavours to develop.
5. When ready to serve, garnish with the parsley.

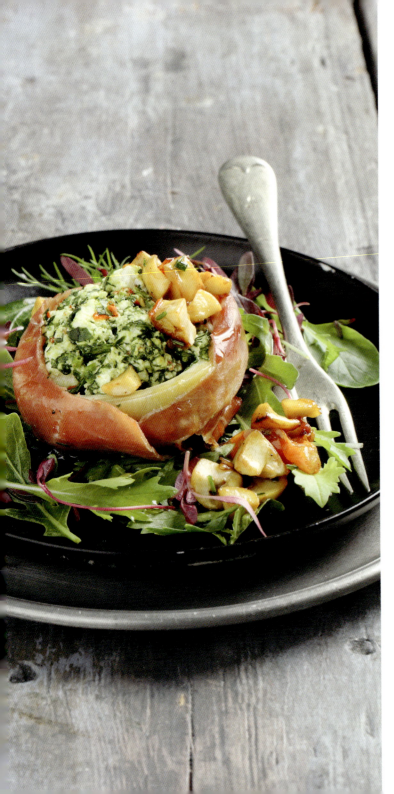

ARTICHOKE CUPCAKES

ARTICHOKE BOTTOMS CREATE THE PERFECT BASE FOR THESE CUPCAKES AND THE PARMA HAM, ONCE COOKED, IS DELICIOUSLY CRISPY. PEPPADEWS ADD PIQUANCY TO THE CREAMY FILLING AND GIVE IT A SOUTH AFRICAN TWIST.

$^1/_3$ cup ricotta cheese
1 Tbsp chopped fresh dill
$^3/_4$ cup finely chopped spinach
3 Peppadews, finely chopped
4 artichoke bottoms
2–4 slices Parma ham, halved lengthways
a little olive oil for frying

$^1/_2$ cup chopped mushrooms
3 cherry tomatoes, finely chopped
$^1/_4$ tsp minced garlic
salt and pepper to taste
fresh greens for serving

1. Preheat the oven to 180°C.
2. Combine the ricotta cheese, dill, spinach and Peppadews.
3. Spoon this mixture into the artichoke bottoms, then wrap the ham around the artichokes.
4. In a pan, heat the olive oil and fry the mushrooms, tomatoes and garlic until the mushrooms soften.
5. Season with salt and pepper. Set aside.
6. Arrange the filled and wrapped artichokes on a baking tray and bake for about 15 minutes or until the ham is crispy.
7. To serve, transfer each artichoke cupcake onto a plate on a bed of fresh greens. Spoon the mushroom mixture around.

BUTTER BEANS & CHORIZO

CHORIZO IS A SAUSAGE OF SPANISH ORIGIN, MADE OF COARSELY GROUND PORK AND HIGHLY SEASONED WITH GARLIC AND CHILLI. IT PAIRS WELL WITH THE BUTTER BEANS TO CREATE A SPICY, GARLICKY STARTER, OVERFLOWING WITH FLAVOUR.

150g spicy chorizo
1 x 410g can butter beans, drained and rinsed
½–1 tsp smoked paprika
¼ cup white wine vinegar
2 Tbsp Old Brown sherry
2 cloves garlic, minced
juice of 2 lemons
1–2 Tbsp chopped fresh mint for garnishing

1. Slice the chorizo into 0.5cm-thick slices and then into half-moons.
2. Fry in a pan until starting to crisp.
3. Add the butter beans to the pan and stir.
4. Mix together the paprika, vinegar, sherry, garlic and lemon juice.
5. Pour over the chorizo and beans, coating well.
6. Simmer gently until the vinegar and sherry have evaporated.
7. Serve warm, garnished with the mint.

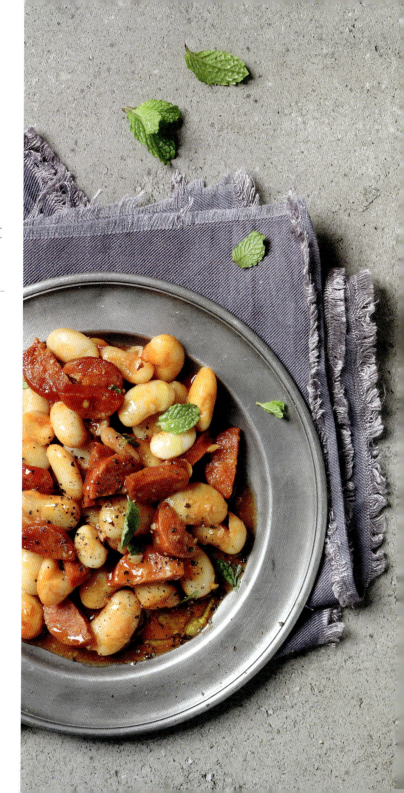

STUFFED LONG PEPPERS

STUFFED VEGETABLES ARE POPULAR ALL AROUND THE MEDITERRANEAN, SO WHY NOT CONTINUE THE TRADITION HERE IN SOUTH AFRICA? RICOTTA MAKES THE PERFECT STUFFING AS IT HOLDS ITS SHAPE DURING COOKING AND SOFTENS WITHOUT MELTING OR OOZING INTO A MESS LIKE MANY OTHER CHEESES.

2 long sweet red peppers
2 Tbsp chopped fresh dill
½ tsp crushed garlic
1 cup crumbled ricotta
salt and pepper to taste
a handful of fresh thyme
2 Tbsp fresh lemon juice

1. Arrange the peppers on a baking tray and place under the grill. Keep turning until the skin has blackened on all sides.
2. Transfer the peppers into a sealable bag for approximately 10 minutes, then remove and peel.
3. Carefully slit each pepper along one side, then remove the pips.
4. In a bowl, mix together the dill, garlic and ricotta cheese. Season liberally with salt and pepper. Use your fingers to crumble the mixture together.
5. Preheat the oven to 180°C.
6. Carefully spoon the mixture into the peppers, closing the slit.
7. Sprinkle the thyme over the base of the baking tray, arrange the peppers on top and place in the centre of the oven. Bake for 20 minutes.
8. When ready, drizzle the lemon juice over the peppers, cut into smaller portions and serve immediately.

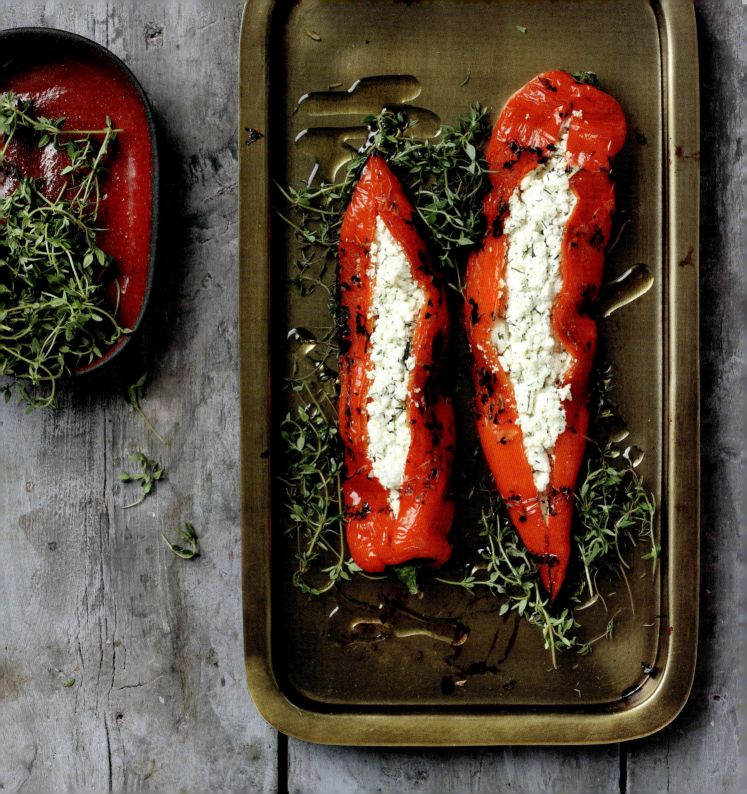

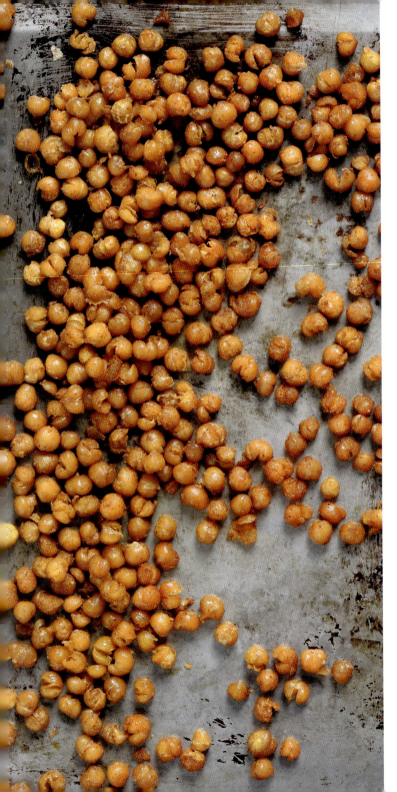

ROASTED CHICKPEAS

CHICKPEAS, ALSO KNOWN AS GARBANZO BEANS, ARE EXCELLENT FOR WEIGHT LOSS DIETS OWING TO THEIR HIGH FIBRE CONTENT AND LOW GI. THEY ARE ALSO A MAJOR INGREDIENT IN MANY MIDDLE EASTERN DISHES, SUCH AS HUMMUS, FALAFELS AND CURRIES. SIMPLY ROASTED WITH SOME SPICES, THEY MAKE THE PERFECT SNACK.

---

1 x 410g can chickpeas, drained and rinsed
2 Tbsp olive oil
¼ tsp cayenne pepper
¼ tsp paprika
2 tsp salt

1. Preheat the oven to 180°C.
2. Pat the chickpeas dry and drizzle the olive oil over them.
3. Mix together the cayenne pepper, paprika and salt.
4. Add the spice mixture to the oiled chickpeas, coating them well. Spread out on a baking tray.
5. Bake in the oven for about 20 minutes, turning them occasionally.
6. Finally, place them under the grill for 5 minutes to crisp.

CUCUMBER, CHEESE & FIG MORSELS

IDEALLY, FRESH FIGS ARE BEST, BUT THEY ARE IN SEASON FOR ONLY A SHORT WHILE, SO IT'S FINE TO USE DRIED FIGS ONCE THE SEASON IS OVER. FIGS ARE SURPRISINGLY HIGH IN BETA-CAROTENE, WHICH IS NEEDED FOR GOOD EYESIGHT, AND THEY'RE A GREAT SOURCE OF ENERGY. THE COOL FRESHNESS OF THE CUCUMBER PROVIDES THE BUILDING BLOCK FOR THE TANGY GOAT'S MILK CHEESE AND SWEET FIG, WHILE THE PISTACHIOS ADD CRUNCH.

80g goat's milk cheese, sliced into rounds
3−4 fresh figs or dried figs or dried dates, sliced
   into rounds
1−2 Tbsp roughly chopped pistachios
¼ cucumber, sliced into 0.5−1cm rounds
honey for drizzling (optional)

1. Place the goat's milk cheese rounds on top of the fig rounds.
2. Sprinkle the pistachios on top of the cheese.
3. Grill the cheese and fig stacks in the oven until the cheese just starts to soften.
4. Place the stacks on top of the cucumber rounds.
5. Drizzle with honey (if using).

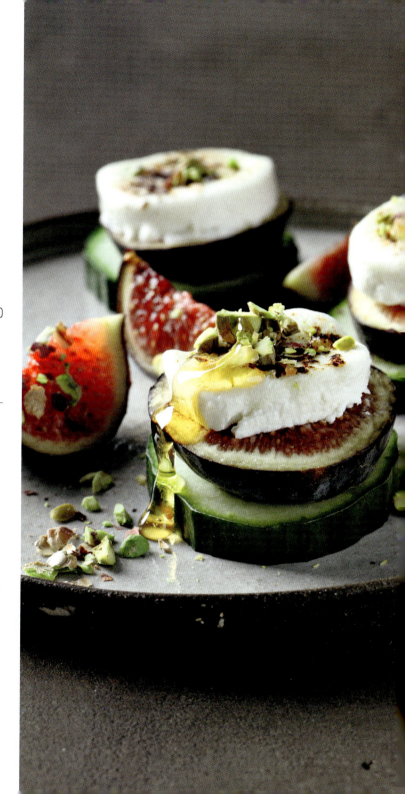

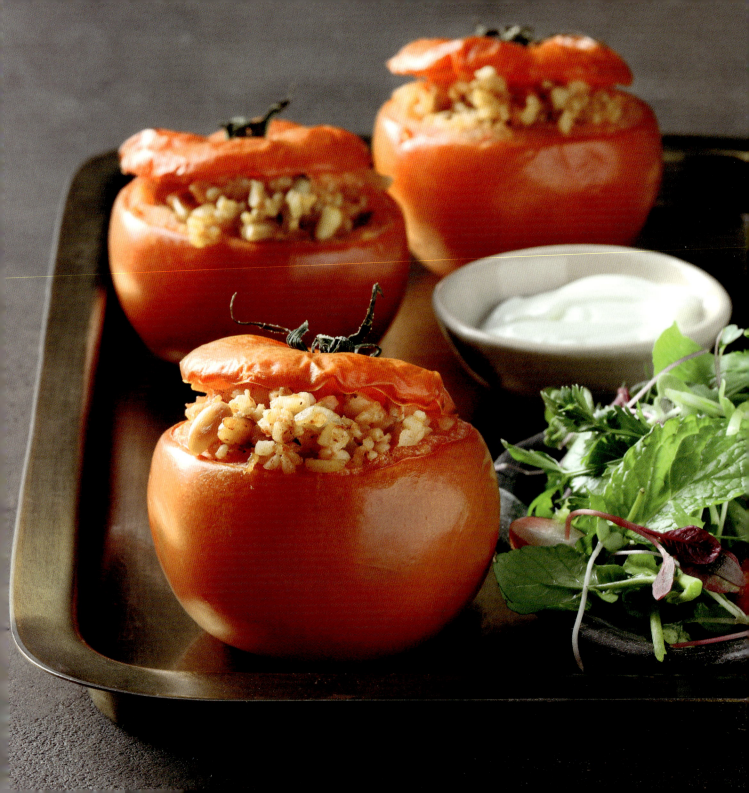

STUFFED TOMATOES

ORIGINATING IN THE SOUTH AMERICAN ANDES NEAR MODERN-DAY PERU, TOMATOES ARE THE FRUIT OF THE TOMATO PLANT. BOTANICALLY THEY'RE CLASSIFIED AS A FRUIT AND NOT A VEGETABLE BECAUSE THEY HAVE SEEDS AND GROW FROM A FLOWERING PLANT. BUT WHATEVER YOU CALL THEM, TOMATOES ARE AN INTEGRAL PART OF MEDITERRANEAN CUISINE. STUFFED TOMATOES ARE EITHER SERVED ON THEIR OWN AS A STARTER OR AS PART OF A LARGER SPREAD WITH OTHER MEZE.

4 large tomatoes
1½ cups water
½ cup bulgur wheat
½ cup chopped onion
a splash of olive oil
1 cup chopped mushrooms
2 Tbsp chopped seedless raisins

4 Tbsp roasted pine nuts
½ tsp ground cinnamon
¼ tsp dried mint
2 Tbsp tomato paste
2 Tbsp water (if necessary)
plain yoghurt for serving
fresh mint leaves for garnishing

1. Preheat the oven to 170°C.
2. Slice the tops off the tomatoes, but reserve for later use. Carefully scoop out the pulp but take care not to break through the skin.
3. Bring the water to the boil in a saucepan, add the bulgur wheat and allow to simmer for approximately 15 minutes or until all the liquid has been absorbed and the wheat is soft.
4. In a separate pan, gently sauté the chopped onion in olive oil until softened.
5. Add the mushrooms and continue to sauté until the mushrooms have softened.
6. Mix the bulgur wheat, and mushroom and onion mixture together.
7. Stir in the raisins, pine nuts, cinnamon, mint and tomato paste until well mixed. (If it's very dry, add the 2 tablespoons of water.)
8. Spoon the mixture into the hollowed tomatoes, filling them to the brim.
9. Arrange the stuffed tomatoes in an ovenproof dish, then pour water in to reach halfway up the tomatoes.
10. Place the tops of the tomatoes back on top and bake in the oven for about 15 minutes.
11. Serve with a dollop of yoghurt and garnish with mint.

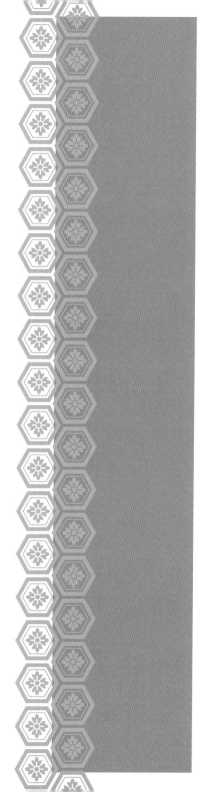

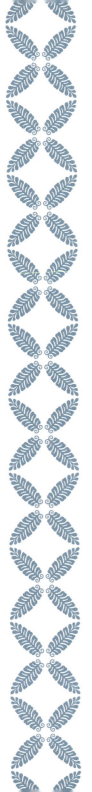

BRINJAL WITH FETA & POMEGRANATES

WE OFTEN ASSOCIATE GRILLED CHEESE WITH ADDED CALORIES, BUT FETA KEEPS THE CALORIE INTAKE AS LOW AS POSSIBLE AND PEOPLE WHO ARE LACTOSE INTOLERANT CAN STILL ENJOY THE CREAMINESS OF THIS DISH IF THEY USE FETA MADE FROM GOAT'S OR SHEEP'S MILK. AND NOT ONLY IS THE BRINJAL TASTY, BUT IT ALSO PROVIDES HEALTH BENEFITS SUCH AS BEING RICH IN BIOFLAVONOIDS – IMPORTANT FOR A HEALTHY HEART.

2 large brinjals
4 Tbsp olive oil
2 cups crumbled feta
4–6 Tbsp pomegranate arils
chopped fresh parsley for garnishing

1. Preheat the oven to 180°C.
2. Cut the brinjals in half lengthways and score the flesh.
3. Brush the olive oil over the scored flesh, then bake the brinjals in the oven for about 20 minutes.
4. Sprinkle the feta on top of each brinjal half.
5. Grill the brinjal halves in the oven until the feta starts to melt.
6. Remove, sprinkle the pomegranate arils over the top, along with a sprinkling of parsley.
7. Serve immediately.

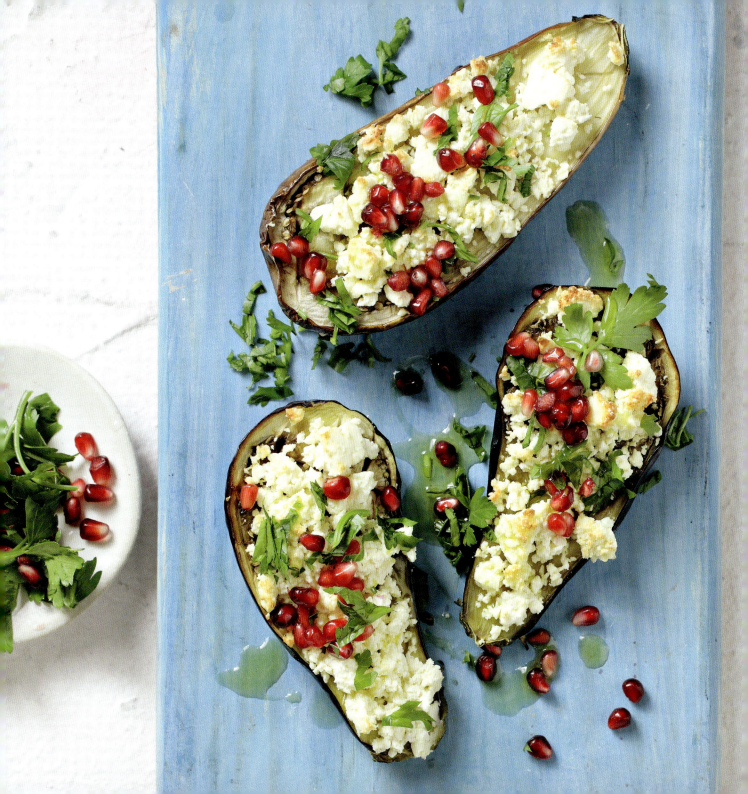

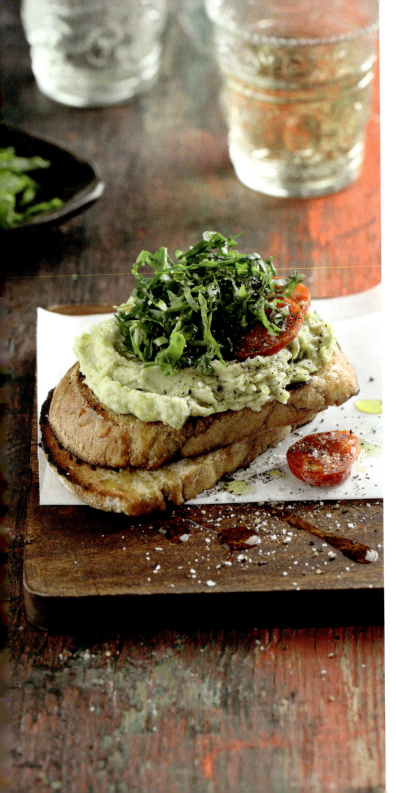

LEEK PURÉE ON RYE

BUTTER BEANS ARE HIGHLY ALKALISING AND A USEFUL SOURCE OF POTASSIUM. BEST OF ALL THOUGH, THEY MAKE A GREAT ACCOMPANIMENT IN A DIP OR PURÉE DUE TO THEIR SOFT, FLOURY TEXTURE. BLENDED HERE WITH LEEKS, THEY'RE PERFECT ON SOME HEALTHY RYE, BUT THIS PURÉE CAN BE USED IN ANY NUMBER OF WAYS.

½ Tbsp olive oil
1 cup chopped leeks
½ cup butter beans
salt and pepper to taste
2 slices rye bread
1 clove garlic, finely sliced
¾ cup finely shredded spinach leaves
¼ cup sliced and fried chorizo

1. In a touch of the olive oil, sauté the leeks until softened, but not browned.
2. Purée the cooked leeks and butter beans together, then season with salt and pepper.
3. Cut the rye slices into quarters then fry them in half a teaspoon of the olive oil and some of the garlic until starting to crisp.
4. Mix together the spinach leaves with the rest of the garlic.
5. Spread the purée thickly onto the fried rye slices, add some shredded spinach and a slice of chorizo.

FLAVOURED MUSHROOMS

MORE OFTEN THAN NOT, MUSHROOMS ARE ADDED TO A STEW
OR ARE MERELY ONE OF MANY OTHER INGREDIENTS IN A DISH.
BUT HERE THEY ARE THE STAR OF THE SHOW. WITH A TOUCH
OF GARLIC AND A SPLASH OF SHERRY VINEGAR
AS ACCOMPANIMENTS, THEIR BEAUTIFUL GOLDEN COLOUR
SHINES THROUGH.

---

1 Tbsp olive oil
125g white mushrooms, roughly chopped
125g brown mushrooms, roughly chopped
1 clove garlic, crushed
1 Tbsp sherry vinegar
1 tsp chopped fresh thyme
a pinch of salt

1. Heat the oil in a pan until quite hot.
2. Add the mushrooms to the pan, coating well with the oil.
3. Do not stir until the mushrooms release all their liquid and turn a golden colour.
4. Reduce the heat, then add the garlic, vinegar and thyme and cook until the vinegar has evaporated.
5. Remove from the heat and season with a pinch of salt.
6. Serve warm or at room temperature. Garnish as desired.

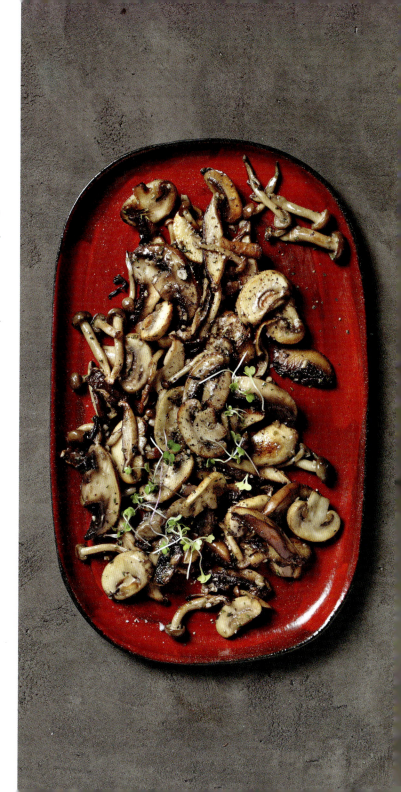

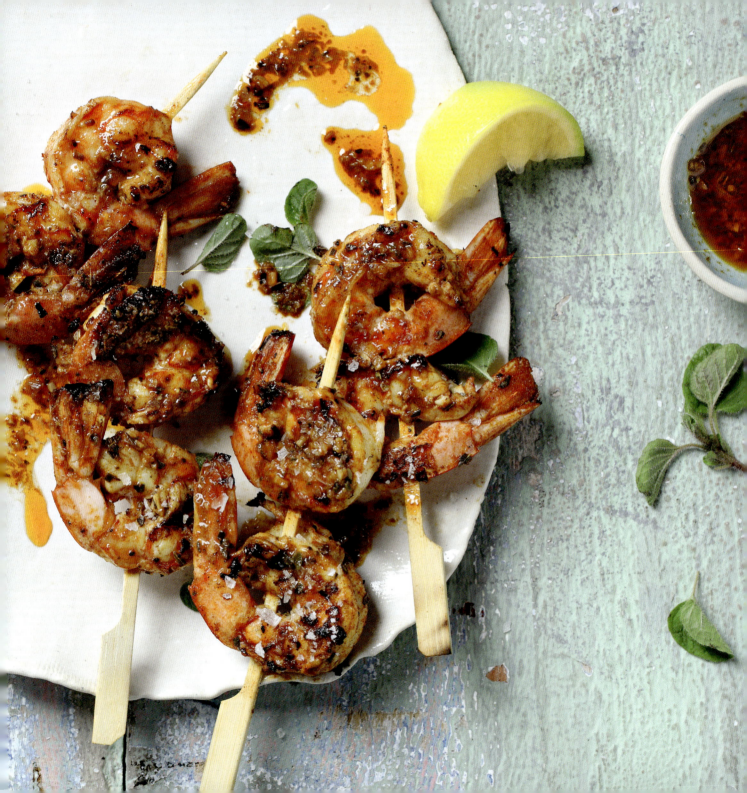

SPANISH PRAWNS

WHAT A TASTY LITTLE SNACK THIS IS! THE SMOKED PAPRIKA IS SPAIN AT ITS BEST, WITH CUMIN AND ORIGANUM THE PERFECT PARTNERS. MARINATING ALLOWS THE MEAT TO SOAK UP ALL THE FLAVOURS, YIELDING SUCCULENT AND DELICIOUS PRAWNS. FEEL FREE TO COOK THEM ON AN OPEN FLAME AS THIS WILL ADD A TOUCH OF SMOKINESS TO THE FLAVOUR.

½ tsp smoked paprika
1 clove garlic, finely chopped
½ tsp ground cumin
½ tsp dried origanum
1 Tbsp olive oil
2 Tbsp lemon juice
200g fresh prawns with tails, shelled and deveined
wooden skewers
½ lemon for serving

1. In a bowl, mix together the paprika, garlic, cumin, origanum, olive oil and lemon juice.
2. Add the prawns, coat well with the mixture and refrigerate for about 1 hour.
3. Thread a few prawns onto each skewer.
4. Heat a griddle pan, add a touch of oil and fry the skewered prawns until cooked.
5. Squeeze the juice of the ½ lemon over the prawn skewers and serve.

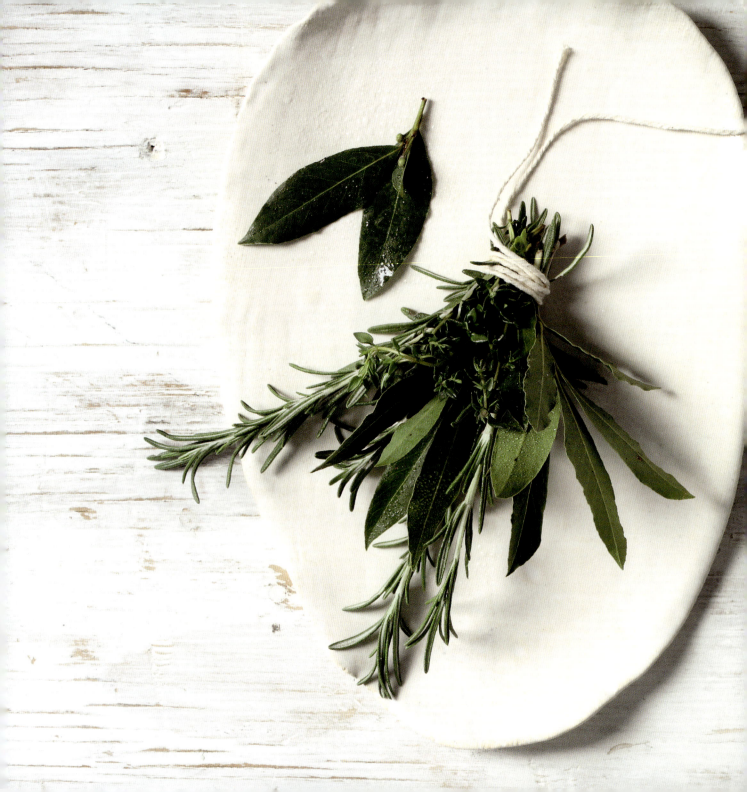

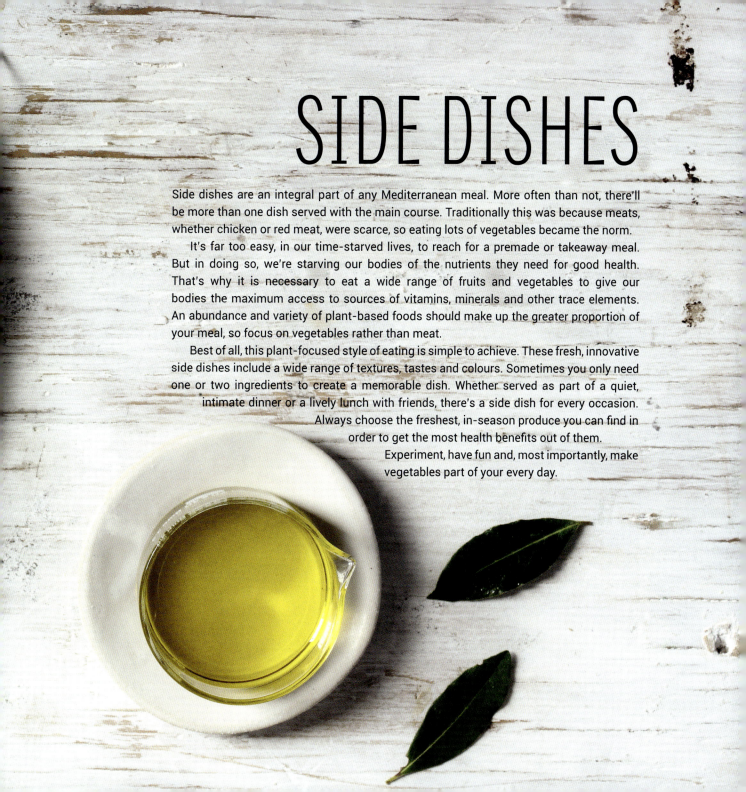

SIDE DISHES

Side dishes are an integral part of any Mediterranean meal. More often than not, there'll be more than one dish served with the main course. Traditionally this was because meats, whether chicken or red meat, were scarce, so eating lots of vegetables became the norm.

It's far too easy, in our time-starved lives, to reach for a premade or takeaway meal. But in doing so, we're starving our bodies of the nutrients they need for good health. That's why it is necessary to eat a wide range of fruits and vegetables to give our bodies the maximum access to sources of vitamins, minerals and other trace elements. An abundance and variety of plant-based foods should make up the greater proportion of your meal, so focus on vegetables rather than meat.

Best of all, this plant-focused style of eating is simple to achieve. These fresh, innovative side dishes include a wide range of textures, tastes and colours. Sometimes you only need one or two ingredients to create a memorable dish. Whether served as part of a quiet, intimate dinner or a lively lunch with friends, there's a side dish for every occasion. Always choose the freshest, in-season produce you can find in order to get the most health benefits out of them. Experiment, have fun and, most importantly, make vegetables part of your every day.

MOROCCAN CARROTS

THIS QUICK-AND-EASY DISH COMBINES SOME SPICY FLAVOURS TO COMPLEMENT THE CRUNCHY CARROTS.
THE ADDITION OF POMEGRANATE ADDS A FURTHER BURST OF COLOUR.

2 Tbsp olive oil
2 Tbsp honey
¼ tsp ground cinnamon
¼ tsp paprika
¼ tsp turmeric
juice of 1 lemon
salt and pepper to taste
250g carrots, peeled and julienned
3 Tbsp chopped fresh coriander
1 Tbsp pomegranate arils

1. Preheat the oven to 180°C.
2. Mix together the olive oil, honey, cinnamon, paprika, turmeric, lemon juice, and salt
   and pepper.
3. Toss the carrots in the mixture and arrange on a baking tray. Bake for 10–15 minutes
   or until just cooked, but not too soft.
4. Scatter over the coriander and pomegranate arils.
5. Serve cold or at room temperature.

THYME-FLAVOURED BABY LEEKS

LEEKS, ALONG WITH GARLIC AND ONIONS, ARE PART OF THE VEGETABLE GENUS ALLIUM. ALTHOUGH THEIR TASTE IS GENTLER AND SWEETER THAN ONIONS, THEY STILL RETAIN MANY OF THE HEALTH-PROMOTING NUTRIENTS FOUND IN THEIR MORE ROBUSTLY FLAVOURED COUNTERPARTS. THE WORD 'ALLIUM' ORIGINATES FROM THE GREED WORD FOR GARLIC.

500g baby leeks
10 sprigs of fresh thyme
¼ cup olive oil
2 Tbsp white wine
salt and pepper to taste
½ Tbsp chopped fresh parsley

1. Preheat the oven to 180°C.
2. Arrange the leeks snugly in a baking dish.
3. Tuck the thyme sprigs in between and around the leeks.
4. Pour over the olive oil and white wine.
5. Cover with aluminium foil and bake for 45 minutes.
6. Remove the foil and continue to bake for another 15 minutes.
7. Season to taste, scatter the parsley over and serve.

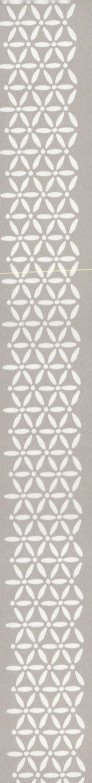

BABY MARROWS & BACON WITH PESTO

ALTHOUGH WE REFER TO THIS SUMMER SQUASH AS 'BABY MARROW', IN EUROPE IT'S MORE COMMONLY KNOWN AS ZUCCHINI OR COURGETTE. IT'S VERY LOW IN CALORIES AND CONTAINS NO SATURATED FATS OR CHOLESTEROL. THE SKIN IS ALSO A HEALTHY SOURCE OF DIETARY FIBRE.

4 Tbsp chopped bacon
450g baby marrows, sliced on the diagonal
olive oil for grilling
1 Tbsp toasted sesame seeds
salt and pepper to taste
2 Tbsp basil pesto
2 Tbsp double thick plain yoghurt

1. Cook the bacon (in a frying pan or microwave) until crispy.
2. Grill the baby marrows in a griddle pan with a little olive oil until griddle lines appear on the slices. Remove and place on a platter.
3. Scatter the bacon bits on top.
4. Finally, scatter the sesame seeds over and season to taste.
5. Mix the basil pesto and yoghurt together.
6. Serve the baby marrows hot or at room temperature, with the pesto mixture on the side.

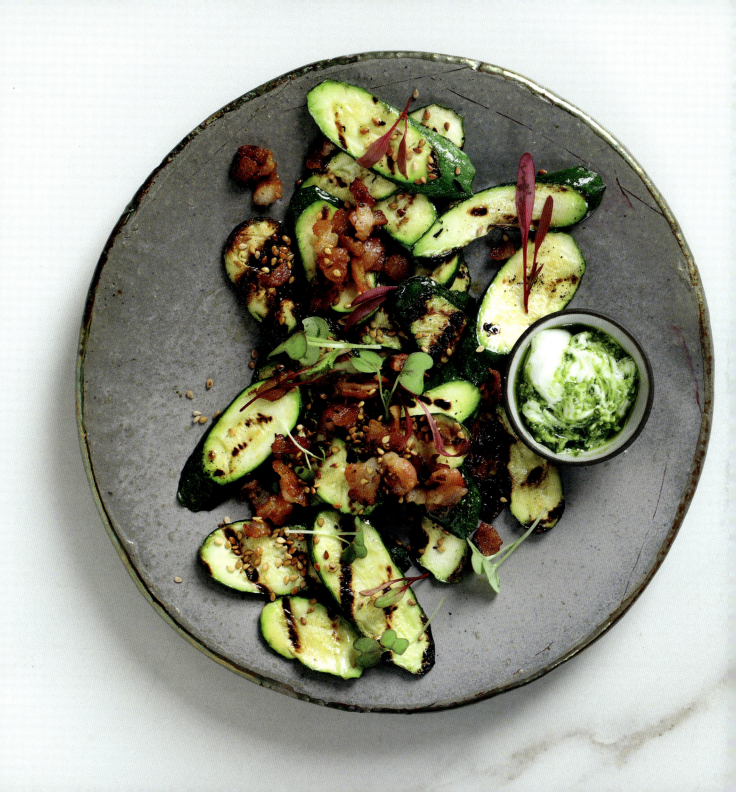

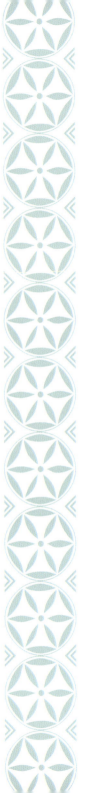

SUGAR SNAP PEAS WITH TARATOR SAUCE

IN TURKEY, 'TARATOR' MEANS A SAUCE MADE WITH WALNUTS, WHILE IN OTHER MIDDLE EASTERN COUNTRIES IT'S MADE WITH SESAME. EITHER WAY, THIS TASTY SAUCE IS THE PERFECT ACCOMPANIMENT TO SUGAR SNAP PEAS, ADDING A NUTTY FLAVOUR.

½ cup chopped walnuts plus 2 Tbsp for garnishing
½ tsp minced garlic
¼ cup lemon juice
3 Tbsp water
300−400g sugar snap peas
½ red onion, sliced
salt and pepper to taste

1. In a blender, purée the half a cup of walnuts, garlic, lemon juice and water. Add a little more water if the tarator sauce is too thick.
2. In a pot of boiling water, cook the peas for about 1 minute. Remove and refresh in ice-cold water to retain the green colour.
3. Coat the peas with the sauce and stir in the onion slices. Season to taste.
4. Transfer the peas to a platter and garnish with the walnuts.
5. Serve at room temperature or chilled.

FENNEL *LIMONE*

FENNEL WAS REVERED BY THE ANCIENT GREEKS AND ROMANS FOR ITS CULINARY AND MEDICINAL PROPERTIES AND IT EVEN APPEARED IN GREEK MYTHOLOGY AS THE MEANS BY WHICH KNOWLEDGE WAS PASSED FROM THE GODS ON OLYMPUS TO MAN. ITS HEAVENLY, AROMATIC TASTE IS ENHANCED WITH THE ADDITION OF LEMON.

---

2 large fennel bulbs, sliced
1 lemon, sliced
¼ cup olive oil
salt and pepper to taste
fennel fronds for garnishing

1. Preheat the oven to 180°C.
2. Arrange the fennel and lemon slices in a baking dish and pour over the olive oil.
3. Season with salt and pepper.
4. Cover with aluminium foil and bake for 1 hour.
5. Remove the foil and continue to bake for another 30 minutes or until all the liquid has been absorbed and the fennel edges have started to brown.
6. Garnish with the fennel fronds.
7. Serve hot or at room temperature.

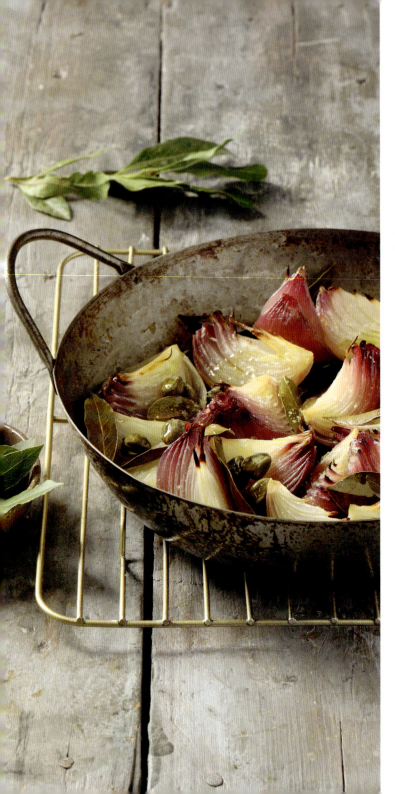

RED ONIONS
WITH CAPERS

THIS DISH CAN BE POPPED INTO THE OVEN AND LEFT TO CREATE ITS OWN MAGIC WHILE YOU DO OTHER THINGS. THE ONIONS BECOME DELICIOUSLY CARAMELISED AND THE CAPERS ARE PERFECT LITTLE BUNDLES OF EXTRA FLAVOUR.

4 red onions, quartered
6–8 dried bay leaves
¼ cup olive oil
1 tsp red wine vinegar
20 capers

1. Preheat the oven to 180°C.
2. Slice the onion quarters into 0.5cm-thick wedges.
3. Arrange the onions snugly in a baking dish and tuck the bay leaves in between the wedges.
4. Pour over the olive oil and vinegar, then cover the dish with aluminium foil.
5. Bake for 45 minutes then remove the foil, add the capers and bake for another 20 minutes.
6. Serve hot or at room temperature.

PARMESAN MUSHROOMS

WHAT COULD BE MORE COMFORTING THAN CREAMY MUSHROOMS? BEST OF ALL, THE CALORIES ARE REDUCED BECAUSE YOGHURT IS SUBSTITUTED FOR CREAM. SHERRY VINEGAR IS A COMPLEX VINEGAR, FULL OF NUTTY FLAVOURS, SO I LOVE USING IT TO ENHANCE THE INTENSITY OF THIS DISH.

300–400g button mushrooms, quartered
¼ cup olive oil
¼ tsp dried origanum
1 Tbsp sherry vinegar
½ tsp minced garlic
salt and pepper to taste
1 Tbsp plain yoghurt
Parmesan shavings

1. In a covered saucepan, sauté the mushrooms in the olive oil over a high heat for approximately 5 minutes.
2. Remove the lid, lower the heat by half and allow the liquid to reduce and the mushrooms to turn golden-brown.
3. Add the origanum, vinegar, garlic, and salt and pepper and continue to sauté until the vinegar has evaporated.
4. Before serving, stir in the yoghurt and scatter the Parmesan shavings over the top. Garnish with fresh herbs if you like.

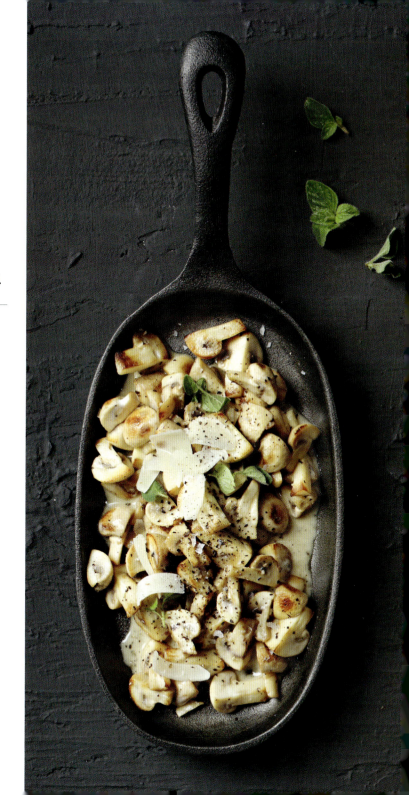

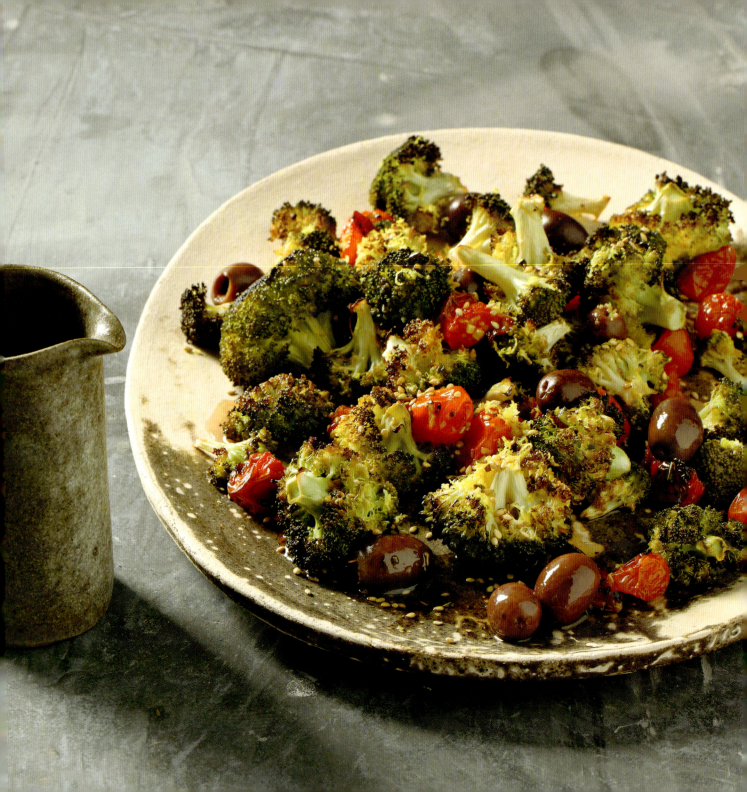

BROCCOLI, TOMATOES & OLIVES

QUINTESSENTIAL MEDITERRANEAN FOOD COLOURS – RIPE RED TOMATOES, GRASS GREEN BROCCOLI AND BROODING BLACK OLIVES – COME TOGETHER IN A RAINBOW DISH THAT IS HEALTHY AND SATISFYING.

3 cups bite-sized broccoli florets
1 cup halved cherry or rosa tomatoes
1 clove garlic, minced
juice of ½ lemon
2 Tbsp olive oil
15 pitted black olives
1 tsp grated lemon zest
1 tsp toasted sesame seeds
chilli flakes (optional)

DRESSING
2 Tbsp olive oil
½ tsp red wine vinegar
¼ tsp honey
¼ tsp dried origanum

1. Preheat the oven to 180°C.
2. Toss the broccoli, tomatoes, garlic, lemon juice and olive oil together, coating well.
3. Spread the broccoli and tomatoes out on a baking tray and bake until the broccoli starts to blacken (7–10 minutes). The broccoli should not be too soft. Leave to cool slightly.
4. Add the olives and mix through.
5. Whisk the dressing ingredients together.
6. Just before serving, pour the dressing over. Sprinkle over the lemon zest, sesame seeds and chilli flakes (if using).
7. Serve warm or at room temperature.

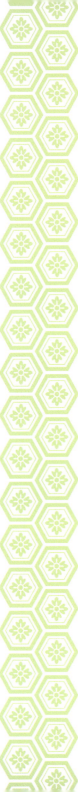

BRINJAL WITH RED PEPPER TOPPING

WHETHER YOU CALL THEM BRINJALS OR AUBERGINES OR EVEN EGGPLANT, THERE'S NO DENYING THEIR DELECTABLE TASTE. I LOVE EATING BRINJALS AND PEPPERS TOGETHER AND HERE THEY MELLOW FOR A WHILE IN OIL, GARLIC AND ORIGANUM – THEIR PERFECT COMPANIONS.

4 brinjals, sliced in 1.5cm-thick rounds
2 Tbsp olive oil
salt and pepper to taste

TOPPING
2 large red peppers
4 tsp red wine vinegar
1 small clove garlic, minced
2½ Tbsp olive oil
½ tsp dried origanum
1 Tbsp roasted pine nuts
2 tsp chopped fresh parsley

1. To prepare the topping, arrange the red peppers on a baking tray and grill in the oven, turning occasionally until they blacken on all sides.
2. Transfer the peppers to a sealable bag and leave them to sweat for about 10 minutes. Once the peppers have cooled, remove them from the bag and peel their skins.
3. Cut the peppers in half and remove all seeds and membranes. Dice the peppers and put into a bowl, along with any of their liquid.
4. Add the vinegar, garlic, olive oil and origanum and stir through. Leave the flavours to combine for at least 30 minutes.
5. To grill the brinjal slices, brush both sides with olive oil and season.
6. Heat a griddle pan until hot then grill the brinjals on both sides until the flesh has softened and the griddle lines are visible.
7. To serve, mix the pine nuts and parsley into the red pepper mixture. Top each slice of brinjal with the topping.

GEM LETTUCE CUPS

THESE INDIVIDUAL LETTUCE LEAVES MAKE THE MOST DELIGHTFUL LITTLE SERVING 'CUPS'. CHOPPING UP ALL THE INGREDIENTS INTO SIMILAR SIZES AND SIMILAR QUANTITIES CREATES A BALANCE OF FLAVOURS AND COLOURS. THE LENTILS OFFER SUBSTANCE WHILE THE DRESSING ADDS SPICE. PERFECT LITTLE GEMS ON A PLATE.

2 cups canned lentils
½ cup cubed carrots
½ cup cubed cucumber
½ cup finely chopped tomato
½ cup finely chopped red onion
10 capers, finely chopped
4 gem lettuce leaves

DRESSING
2 Tbsp olive oil
2 Tbsp Greek yoghurt
½ tsp lemon juice
¼ tsp ground cumin
½ tsp cayenne pepper
1 tsp honey
salt and pepper to taste

1. First make the dressing by mixing all the ingredients together.
2. Combine all the other ingredients, except the lettuce leaves. Pour the dressing over, making sure everything is well coated.
3. Spoon the lentil mixture into the gem lettuce cups.
4. Arrange carefully on a serving platter.

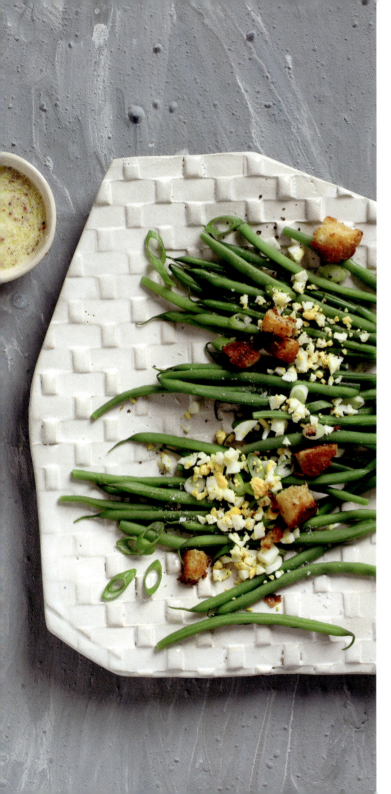

GREEN BEANS & EGGS

SOME ANCIENT CULTS BELIEVED THAT HUMAN SOULS TRAVELLED THROUGH THE STEMS OF BEANS TO THEIR NEXT LIVES, THUS IT WAS FORBIDDEN TO EAT BEANS OR EVEN WALK AMONG THE PLANTS. NOWADAYS, IT'S IMPORTANT TO INCLUDE THEM IN YOUR DIET AS THEY'RE RICH IN NUTRIENTS FOR BOTH YOUR BODY AND THE SOIL, AS THEIR ROOTS ADD NITROGEN INTO THE SOIL RATHER THAN DEPLETING IT.

180g extra fine fresh green beans, stems removed
1 spring onion, finely chopped
1 hard-boiled egg, finely chopped
¼ cup croutons

DRESSING
1 Tbsp olive oil
1 tsp prepared wholegrain mustard
1 Tbsp plain yoghurt
½ tsp water, if necessary
salt and pepper to taste

1. Cook the green beans in salted boiling water until *al dente*. When ready, transfer to a serving bowl.
2. Mix the dressing ingredients together, then pour over the beans.
3. Sprinkle over the spring onion, chopped egg and croutons.
4. Serve either warm or at room temperature.

STUFFED GEM SQUASH

THIS MAKES A GOOD ALTERNATIVE TO THE LARGE STUFFED MARROWS YOU SEE IN MANY MEDITERRANEAN RESTAURANTS AND HOMES. WHEN CHOOSING A SQUASH, IT SHOULD MAKE A HOLLOW SOUND WHEN TAPPED AND THE SKIN SHOULD BE SHINY AND DARK GREEN. THE FLESH IS NORMALLY SWEETER THAN OTHER SQUASH VARIETIES.

2 gem squash, halved and seeds removed
½ cup frozen peas
1 cup roughly chopped baby spinach leaves
1 Tbsp olive oil
⅓ cup crumbled feta
salt and pepper to taste
2 Tbsp stale breadcrumbs, fried

1. Cook the squash in boiling water until tender.
2. Cook the peas separately until softened.
3. In a pan, heat the spinach in the olive oil, until just wilted.
4. Remove from the heat and stir through the peas and feta, then season with salt and pepper.
5. Spoon this mixture into the squash centres and sprinkle the breadcrumbs on top.

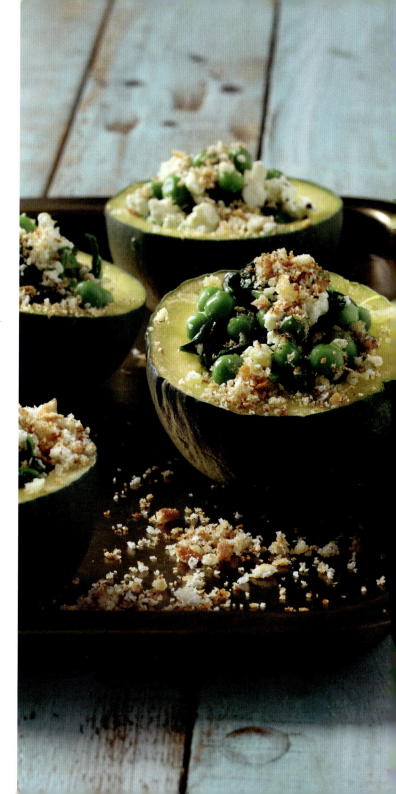

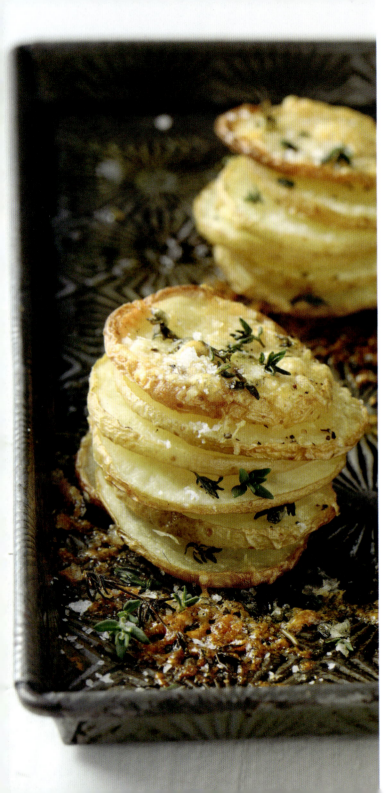

POTATO STACKS

WHO CAN RESIST POTATOES AND CHEESE? NO MATTER HOW MANY OF THESE YOU MAKE, THERE'LL NEVER BE ANY LEFT OVER. PARMESAN IS A RELATIVELY LOW FAT CHEESE, SO IT'S IDEAL TO COMBINE WITH POTATOES TO KEEP THE CALORIES AS LOW AS POSSIBLE. WITH THE ADDITION OF THYME, MEDITERRANEAN FLAVOURS WILL EXPLODE IN YOUR MOUTH.

2 Tbsp olive oil
½ tsp dried or 1 tsp fresh thyme
4 small unpeeled potatoes, finely sliced
coarse salt
grated Parmesan for serving

1. Preheat the oven to 180°C.
2. Combine the olive oil and thyme.
3. Coat each slice of potato with the olive oil mixture.
4. Stack the potato slices one on top of each other, 4–5 slices per stack.
5. Sprinkle salt over the top of each stack.
6. Arrange the stacks on a baking tray and bake for 30–40 minutes or until the edges turn crispy.
7. Once cooked, sprinkle a little Parmesan on top of each stack and place under the grill to melt the cheese.
8. Serve immediately.

CACIK

THIS REFRESHING DISH IS COMMONLY SERVED WITH TURKISH MEALS AS YOGHURT IS CENTRAL TO THEIR DIET. A COLD, CRUNCHY SALAD, IT'S EASY TO WHIP UP AND IS BEST SERVED WITH GRILLED MEATS OR CHICKEN. THE GREEK VERSION OF THIS RECIPE IS CALLED 'TZATZIKI'.

---

4 Tbsp Greek yoghurt
4 Tbsp chopped, peeled cucumber
½ tsp crushed garlic
2 tsp olive oil

1. Mix the ingredients together.
2. Serve chilled.

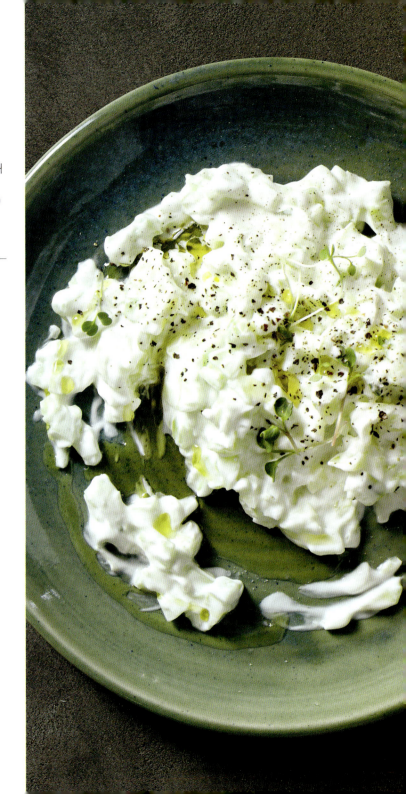

GREEN BEANS
WITH MUSHROOMS

MUSHROOMS ARE IDEAL FOR ABSORBING DELICIOUS SAUCES AND THIS SIDE DISH, EATEN WITH CHICKEN VÉRONIQUE, IS THE PERFECT PARTNER. ANCIENT EGYPTIANS BELIEVED THAT MUSHROOMS GREW BY MAGIC BECAUSE THEY WOULD APPEAR OVERNIGHT. NOT ONLY ARE THEY MAGICAL, BUT THEY'RE HEALTHY TOO, AS A GOOD SOURCE OF VITAMIN D.

170g fresh green beans
4—5 white mushrooms
2 Tbsp olive oil
salt and pepper to taste

1. Sauté the green beans and mushrooms in the oil until just cooked.
2. Season with salt and pepper.

LEEK & BABY MARROW PILAF

MANY TURKISH RECIPES END WITH THE INSTRUCTION 'AND SERVE WITH RICE'. HOWEVER, THE RICE ISN'T SERVED ON THE SAME PLATE BUT IS USUALLY A DISH IN ITSELF AND SERVED SEPARATELY. THERE ARE AS MANY VARIATIONS OF PILAF AS THERE ARE GRAINS OF RICE, BUT GENERALLY IT MEANS THAT THE RICE HAS BEEN COOKED IN STOCK.

---

3 leeks, chopped
3 baby marrows, chopped
olive oil for frying
1 chicken stock cube
3 cups boiling water
½ cup brown rice
salt and pepper to taste
juice of ½ lemon
chopped fresh parsley for garnishing

1. Sauté the leeks and baby marrows in a little heated olive oil until softened.
2. Add the stock cube to the water and boil the rice in the stock until cooked. Drain the rice if necessary.
3. Combine the leeks and baby marrows with the rice, then season with salt and pepper. Squeeze the lemon juice over the rice and stir through.
4. Garnish with the parsley.

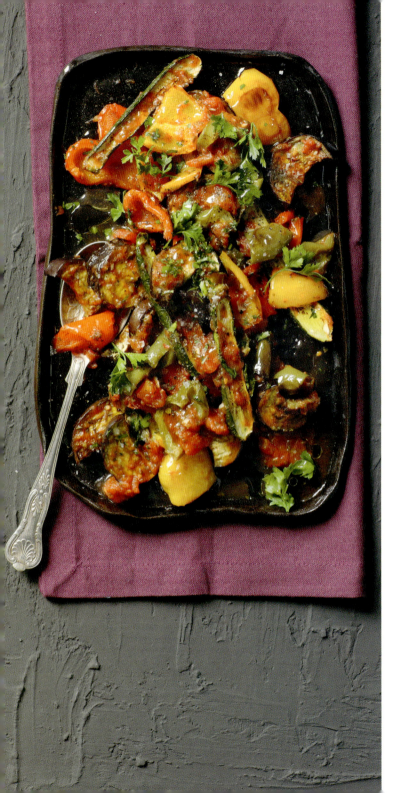

BRIAM (MIXED VEGETABLES)

THIS IS A GREEK FAVOURITE, REDOLENT OF THE AROMAS OF FRESH HERBS AND VEGETABLES. IT SHOWS THE SIMPLICITY OF THEIR CUISINE, TAKING THE SIMPLEST OF INGREDIENTS AND TRANSFORMING THEM INTO A PURE DELIGHT, WITH VERY LITTLE EFFORT. THE DISH FORMS PART OF GREEK CUISINE KNOWN AS *LADERA*, WHICH MEANS DISHES PREPARED WITH OLIVE OIL. USE THE HIGHEST QUALITY OLIVE OIL YOU CAN AFFORD.

1 medium brinjal, sliced into rings
1 green pepper, roughly chopped
1 red pepper, roughly chopped
1 yellow pepper, roughly chopped
4–5 baby marrows, roughly chopped
1 red onion, roughly chopped
olive oil
2 Tbsp chopped fresh dill
2 Tbsp chopped fresh parsley, plus extra for garnishing
1–2 cloves garlic, finely chopped
salt and pepper to taste
$3/4$ cup canned chopped and peeled tomatoes

1. Preheat the oven to 180°C.
2. Arrange the brinjal, peppers, baby marrows and onion on a baking tray and pour over enough olive oil to coat the vegetables.
3. Add the dill, parsley, garlic, salt and pepper and mix well.
4. Add the tomatoes and stir through.
5. Cover the dish with foil and bake for about 90 minutes.
6. Garnish with the extra parsley.

GREEN PEPPER CUPS WITH COOKED *CAPRESE* SALAD

2 green peppers, halved and deseeded
2 Tbsp olive oil
6–8 small tomatoes
6–8 *bocconcini* (small round mozzarella balls)
1 round feta cheese, cubed
a few sprigs of fresh mint leaves
4 Tbsp finely chopped fresh basil or baby
    spinach leaves
salt and pepper to taste
a pinch of dried origanum
a pinch of sugar

1. Preheat the oven to 180°C.
2. Rub the outside of the green peppers with the olive oil.
3. Place the peppers, cut-side side down, on a baking tray and bake for about 15 minutes or until softened.
4. Spoon the tomatoes, *bocconcini*, feta, mint and basil or spinach leaves into the green pepper halves. Season with salt and pepper, then sprinkle over the origanum and sugar and bake in the oven for about 7 minutes or until the cheese starts to melt and the tomatoes soften.

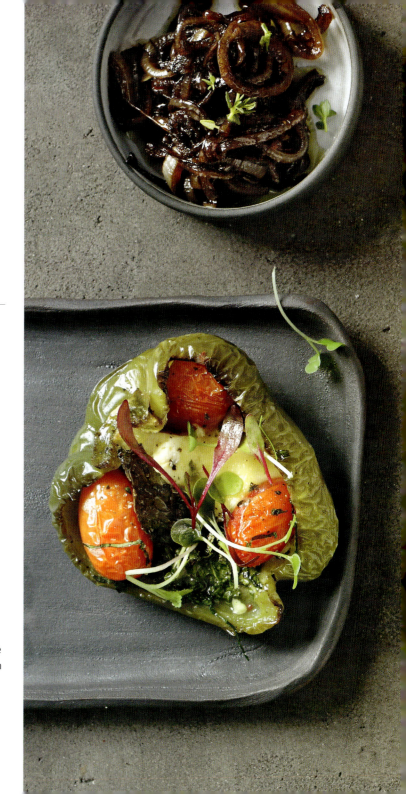

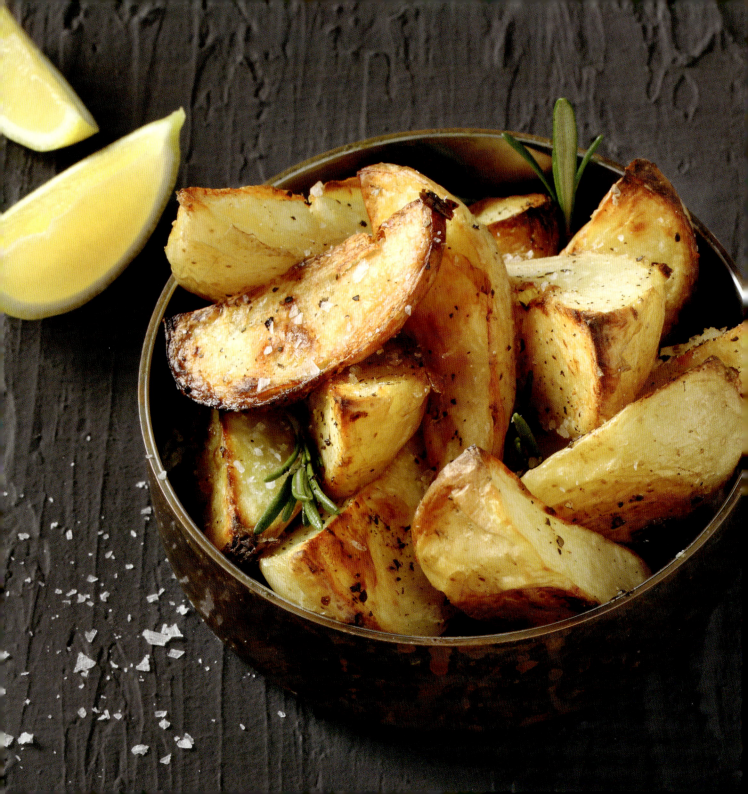

GREEK-STYLE LEMON POTATOES

CRISP MEETS CREAMY IN ONE TASTY MOUTHFUL. THE COMBINATION OF THE SALT, ROSEMARY AND TANGY LEMON IS SIMPLY SUBLIME. BUT DON'T PEEL THE POTATOES AS MANY NUTRIENTS ARE PACKED INTO THAT CRISPY OUTER LAYER. POTATOES HAVE MORE POTASSIUM THAN BANANAS, PROVIDING MORE THAN HALF YOUR NECESSARY DAILY VITAMIN C REQUIREMENT FROM ONE POTATO.

4–5 unpeeled potatoes
olive oil
coarse salt
pepper to taste
2 lemons
2 sprigs of fresh rosemary

1. Boil the potatoes in their jackets until just cooked.
2. Drain and leave them until just cool enough to handle.
3. Cut the potatoes into wedges and rub olive oil all over them.
4. Arrange on a baking tray, season liberally with salt and pepper, squeeze the juice of one lemon over the wedges and scatter the rosemary sprigs over them.
5. Place under the grill until they start to brown.
6. Remove, turn and place under the grill again.
7. Once done, squeeze the juice of the second lemon over the potato wedges and serve immediately.

GREEN PEPPERS WITH CAPERS

THE SPINACH PROVIDES THE FIBRE, GREEN PEPPERS THE MANGANESE AND CAPERS THE VITAMIN K, BUT IT'S REALLY ALL ABOUT THE FLAVOURS. A FEW CAPERS CAN CREATE A BIG, BOLD TASTE WHILE ONLY CONTAINING TWO CALORIES PER TABLESPOON.

2 Tbsp olive oil

3 green peppers, sliced into strips

1 yellow pepper, sliced into strips

4 cloves garlic, sliced

3 Tbsp capers

¼ cup sherry vinegar

1–2 cups baby spinach leaves

1. Heat the olive oil in a pan and fry the peppers. Stir frequently until they are charred.
2. Add the garlic, capers and vinegar and stir through. Keep simmering to allow the vinegar to evaporate.
3. Stir in the baby spinach leaves.
4. Remove when the spinach leaves start to wilt.
5. Serve immediately.

GRILLED ASPARAGUS

SIMPLICITY IS PERFECTION, SO MUCH SO THAT QUEEN NEFERTITI OF EGYPT DECLARED ASPARAGUS TO BE THE FOOD OF THE GODS. CHOOSE THE FRESHEST ASPARAGUS YOU CAN FIND AND ALL THAT IS NEEDED IS A TOUCH OF SEASONING. THE TRUE FLAVOURS OF ASPARAGUS WILL SHINE THROUGH.

225g fresh green baby asparagus
2 Tbsp olive oil
salt and pepper to taste
juice of 1 lemon

1. In a pot of boiling water, blanche the asparagus for 2 minutes.
2. Remove and refresh in cold water.
3. Heat a griddle pan to hot.
4. Sauté the asparagus in the olive oil until they begin to char.
5. Season to taste.
6. Squeeze the lemon juice over the asparagus as soon as you are ready to serve.

ROASTED TOMATOES, CHICKPEAS & SPRING ONION

THIS TASTY SIDE DISH HAS THE SPICY FLAVOURS OF PAPRIKA BALANCING WITH THE SALTINESS OF THE FETA AND THE EARTHINESS OF THE CHICKPEAS, ALL DRAWN TOGETHER IN THE DEEP RED COLOUR OF ROASTED TOMATO. A FEAST FOR THE EYES AS WELL AS THE TASTE BUDS.

1 x 410g can chickpeas, drained
olive oil
1½ cups halved or quartered rosa tomatoes
4 Tbsp sliced spring onions
1 round feta cheese
salt and pepper to taste

1. In a hot pan, dry-fry the chickpeas until they start to harden. Remove and set aside.
2. Add a few drops of olive oil to the pan, then add the tomatoes.
3. Cook the tomatoes until they start to blister. Remove and set aside.
4. Add the spring onions to the pan and cook until softened.
5. In a serving dish, combine the tomatoes, chickpeas and spring onions.
6. Drizzle over some olive oil.
7. Finally, crumble the feta cheese over the top and season with salt and pepper to taste.

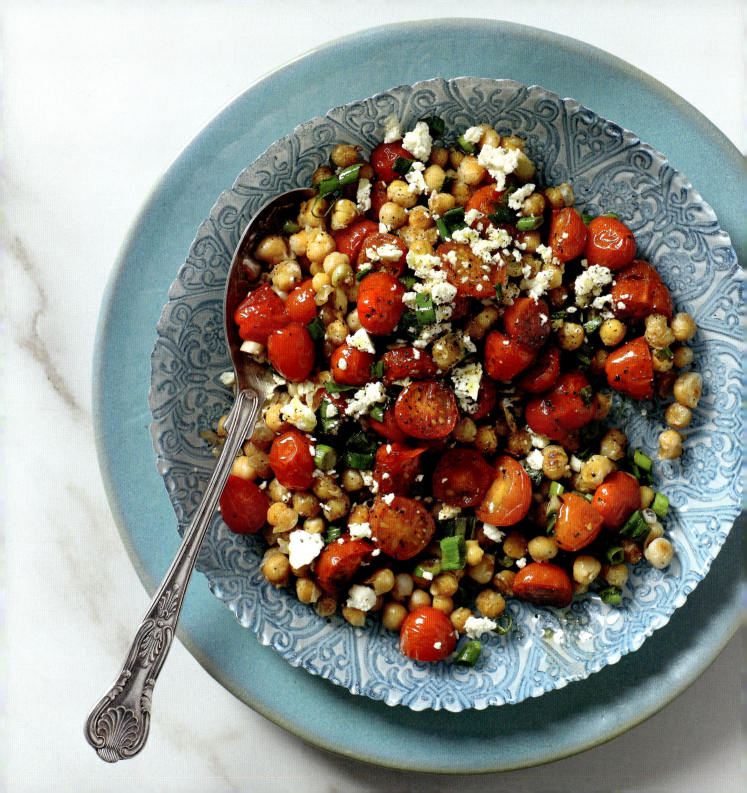

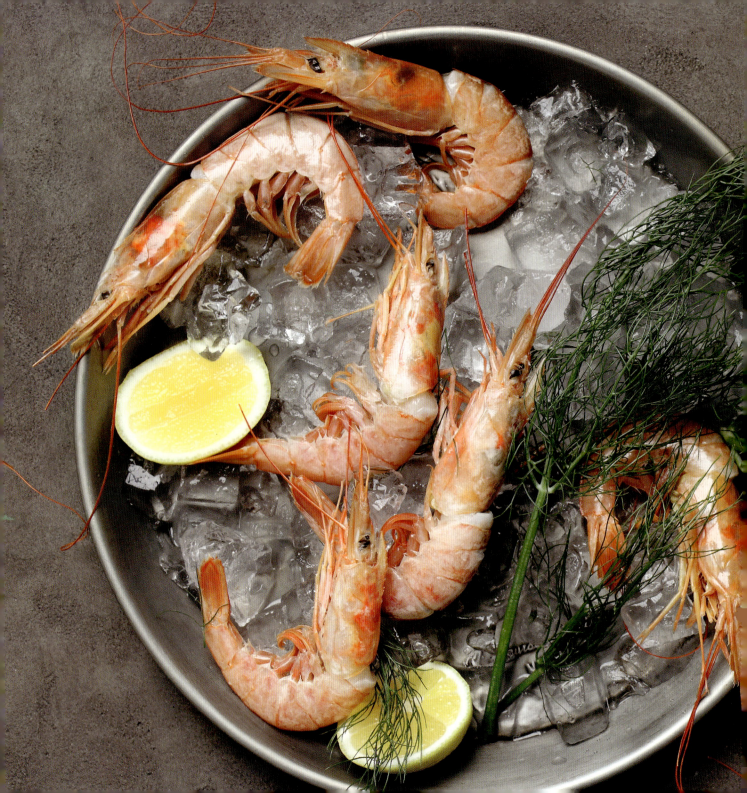

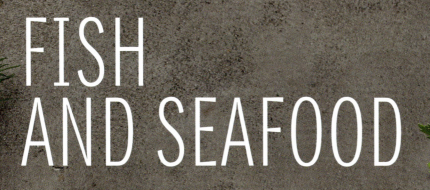

FISH
AND SEAFOOD

Turquoise waters, colourful fishing boats, an abundance of sunshine and romantic sunsets over glittering seas … all images that spring to mind when thinking of the Mediterranean.

In the sea, there is an abundance of fish and seafood. With such a long coastline, it's only natural that they play an important role in the Mediterranean diet. Here in South Africa, we have a wide variety of seafood and fish of our own, though we have to be discerning when selecting the fish we eat as some local fish stocks are coming under pressure. To ensure that you're choosing ethically, consult the latest SASSI list at website: wwfsassi.co.za

Fish and seafood are rich in minerals and nutrients. They are high in protein, low in saturated fat and a rich source of vitamin D and selenium.

The recipes I've selected vary from famous dishes such as paella from Spain to my own individual dishes, such as marinated calamari salad served with the ingredients you'd find in a Caprese salad. They all have a unique Mediterranean charm and evoke the distinctive laid-back lifestyle that seduces us all.

There is a surprising similarity between the seafood and fish that are available in South African waters and along the Mediterranean coast. Shared favourites include prawns, calamari, tuna and hake. But it's also easy to make substitutions. Sea bass, eaten throughout the Mediterranean, is a firm white fish that can be substituted with yellowtail or kabeljou ,while kingklip is a handy substitute for red snapper and grouper.

These fish and seafood dishes are all easy to prepare, with the focus on simplicity and fresh ingredients. I realise, however, that fresh seafood isn't always available. The best way to thaw fish is to leave it in a sealed bag in the fridge to thaw gradually, allowing it to retain texture and flavour. But if you're really pressed for time, place it in a sealed bag, in a pot of cold water for at least 30 minutes.

AMALFI TOMATO TUNA

LEMONS AND FISH ARE PERFECT PARTNERS AND ITALY'S AMALFI COAST IS WELL KNOWN FOR ITS FRAGRANT LEMON GROVES. THE COLOUR COMBINATIONS OF THIS DISH REMIND ME OF THE BRIGHT BEACH UMBRELLAS YOU SEE ALONG THIS MAJESTIC COASTLINE. THE HEALTH BENEFITS OF EATING TUNA ARE CONSIDERABLE AS IT'S RICH IN OMEGA-3 FATTY OIL, HIGH IN PROTEIN AND LIFTS THE BODY'S MAGNESIUM AND POTASSIUM LEVELS. SERVE THE TUNA WITH BABY POTATOES IN THEIR JACKETS.

400–500g tuna steaks
salt and pepper
8–10 baby marrows, finely sliced
   (use a cheese slicer)
2 Tbsp olive oil
8 whole baby potatoes

MARINADE
14 capers
2 Tbsp white wine
juice of 2 lemons
4 Tbsp medium-fat plain yoghurt

SAUCE
8 sun-dried tomatoes, finely chopped
2 cups chopped rosa tomatoes
¼ cup balsamic vinegar
1 tsp finely chopped garlic
¼ cup dry white wine
2 Tbsp chopped fresh basil
¼ cup water (if necessary)

DRESSING FOR POTATOES
4 Tbsp medium-fat plain yoghurt
2 Tbsp tangy mayonnaise
2 Tbsp chopped fresh basil
chopped fresh chives for garnishing

1. For the marinade, place the capers, white wine, lemon juice and yoghurt in a blender and blitz until finely chopped.
2. Season the tuna steaks liberally with pepper and a touch of salt, then place in a sealable bag.
3. Pour the marinade into the bag and toss to ensure that the tuna steaks are well coated.
4. Refrigerate for a minimum of 30 minutes.
5. To prepare the sauce, gently sauté the sun-dried tomatoes, rosa tomatoes, balsamic vinegar, garlic, white wine and basil in a saucepan for about 5 minutes. If it starts to dry out, add the quarter cup of water. Set aside.
6. Place the baby marrows in a pan with 1 tablespoon of the olive oil and sauté until they start to brown.
7. Season with salt and pepper. Set aside, but keep warm.
8. Boil the potatoes until cooked but still firm.
9. To make the dressing, mix together the yoghurt, mayonnaise and basil, then season with salt and pepper.
10. Remove the tuna from the bag (discard the marinade) and sauté in a preheated pan until just done on the outside, but still quite rare on the inside. Remove and keep warm.
11. To serve, arrange some of the baby marrows on each plate, place a tuna steak on top and spoon over some sauce. Add a few baby potatoes to each plate and pour some of the dressing over them, then sprinkle with chives. If you like, you could also serve lemon wedges on the side.

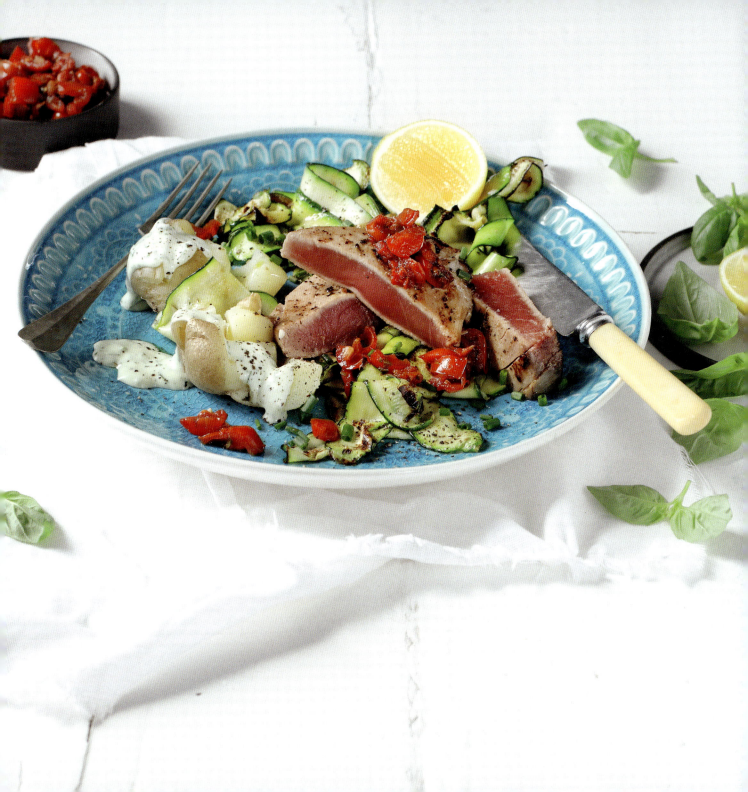

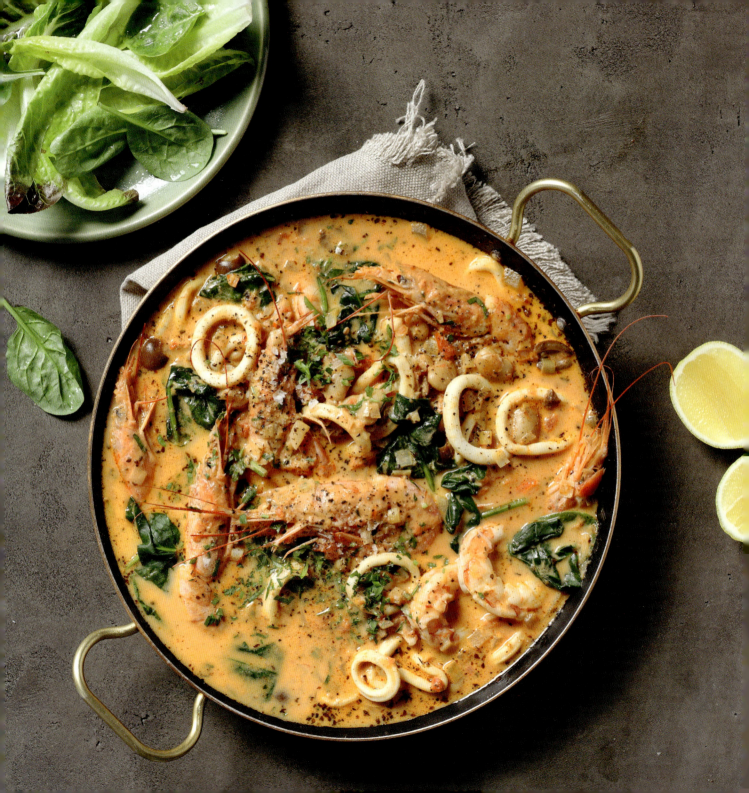

MARSEILLE SEAFOOD STEW

THE FRENCH MAKE A DELICIOUS FISH SOUP CALLED BOUILLABAISSE, WHICH ORIGINATED IN MARSEILLE. THE FISHERMEN WOULD MAKE A STEW FROM THE UNSOLD FISH AT THE END OF THE DAY, BUT THERE ARE MANY VERSIONS. EACH MARSEILLAIS FAMILY AND RESTAURANT ARE CONVINCED THAT THEIRS IS THE AUTHENTIC DISH. THIS RECIPE IS A VERY LOOSE ADAPTATION – MORE A STEW THAN A BROTH – BUT EQUALLY DELICIOUS.

500g calamari rings
2 cups milk
2 cloves garlic, finely sliced
juice of 1 lemon
2 Tbsp olive oil
1 onion, chopped
2 leeks, chopped
2 whole cloves garlic
2 tsp dried mixed herbs

½ tsp smoked paprika
½–1 chilli, finely chopped
½ cup pitted and halved black olives
1 x 410g can butter beans
1 x 400g can chopped tomatoes
grated zest of 1 lemon

200–300g prawns, shelled and deveined
2 cups baby spinach leaves
salt and pepper to taste
4 large cooked, unshelled prawns for garnishing
sprigs of fresh parsley for garnishing

1. Marinate the calamari in the milk, sliced garlic and half the lemon juice for at least 2 hours.
2. Add the olive oil to a large saucepan and gently fry the onion, leeks, whole garlic, mixed herbs, paprika and chilli for a few minutes.
3. Stir in the olives, beans and tomatoes, then simmer for about 5 minutes.
4. Remove the calamari from the marinade and set aside.
5. Pour the marinade into the olive-and-bean mixture, as well as the lemon zest and remaining lemon juice. Allow the sauce to simmer and thicken for 15–20 minutes.
6. Add the shelled prawns, calamari and spinach. Simmer, without stirring, for about 5 minutes or until the calamari is just cooked. (Be careful not to overcook the calamari and prawns.)
7. Season with salt and pepper.
8. To serve, arrange the 4 large unshelled prawns on top and scatter over the parsley.
9. Serve in bowls with brown rice to soak up the sauce and a simple green salad. Or for a more indulgent option, substitute the brown rice with a freshly sliced French baguette.

CHERMOULA FISH SALAD

CHERMOULA IS TRADITIONALLY A MOROCCAN AND TUNISIAN HERB AND SPICE MARINADE USED TO FLAVOUR FISH AND OTHER DISHES. IT'S PERFECT FOR ADDING DELICIOUS FLAVOUR TO KINGKLIP, THE WHITE, DEEP-SEA FISH FOUND IN THE SEAS AROUND SOUTH AFRICA. A SIMILAR FISH CAUGHT OFF MOROCCO AND ALONG THE MEDITERRANEAN COAST IS SEA BASS. IN THIS SALAD THE ORANGE SEGMENTS PROVIDE JUST THE RIGHT COMBINATION OF SWEET 'N SOUR TO CONTRAST DELIGHTFULLY WITH THE SIZZLING FLAVOUR OF THE FIRM-FLESHED FISH – CREATING A PERFECT BALANCE FOR THE PALATE.

400– 500g kingklip, cubed
olive oil for frying
salt
2 oranges, peeled and segmented
2 Tbsp fresh mint
3 spring onions, chopped
1 cup rocket
1 cup mixed salad greens
¼ cup roasted almonds, chopped
1 Tbsp pomegranate arils

CHERMOULA PASTE
2 cloves garlic
½ tsp crushed ginger
¾ cup chopped fresh parsley
¾ cup chopped fresh coriander
3 Tbsp olive oil
2 Tbsp orange juice
1 tsp ground cumin
½ tsp cayenne pepper
½ tsp coriander seeds
⅛ tsp ground cinnamon

DRESSING
¼ cup olive oil
2 Tbsp orange juice
a pinch of ground cinnamon
salt and pepper to taste

1. Blend all the chermoula paste ingredients together.
2. Coat the fish with the paste, then refrigerate for about 1 hour.
3. Heat a little olive oil in griddle pan and fry the fish a few minutes on each side, until cooked. Season the fish with salt.
4. Combine the oranges, mint, spring onions, rocket and salad greens, then arrange on a platter.
5. Place the fish on top of the salad.
6. Whisk the dressing ingredients together and pour over the salad and fish.
7. Finally, scatter the almonds and pomegranate arils over all and serve immediately.

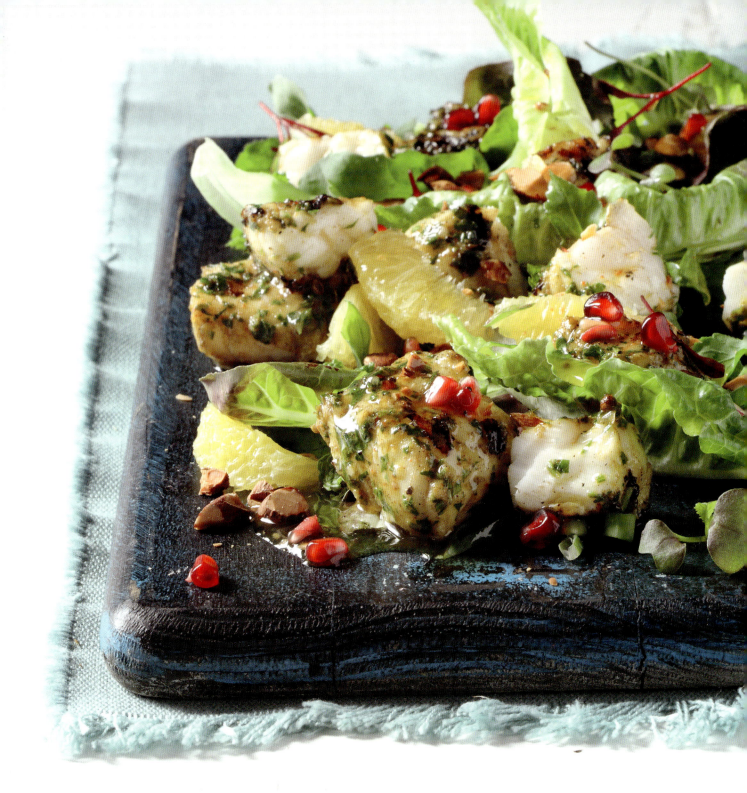

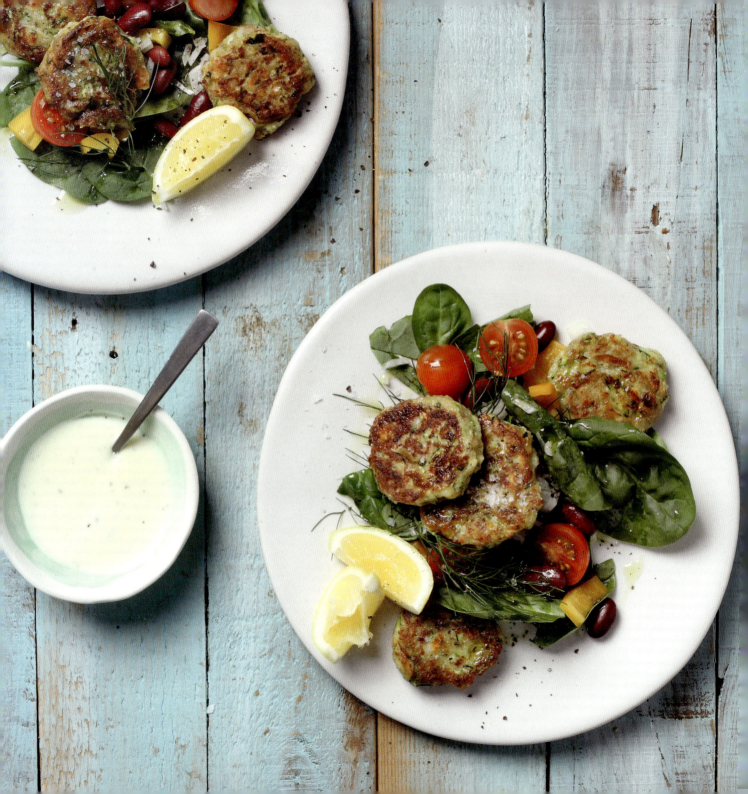

CYCLADIC TUNA CROQUETTES WITH BABY MARROWS

CROQUETTE IS FROM THE FRENCH WORD '*CROQUER*', WHICH MEANS 'TO CRUNCH', A PERFECT DESCRIPTION OF THESE CRUNCHY BALLS OF FLAVOUR. THE CYCLADES ARE A GROUP OF GREEK ISLANDS THAT FORM A CIRCLE AROUND THE SACRED ISLAND OF DELOS. THE CROQUETTES CAN BE EATEN ON THEIR OWN (THE WAY THEY ARE SERVED ON THESE SCENIC ISLANDS) OR AS PART OF A SALAD (MY PREFERENCE) TO CREATE A MORE SUBSTANTIAL MEAL.

1 x 410g can red kidney beans
¼ onion, chopped
½ cup halved cherry tomatoes
½ yellow pepper, chopped
1 cup baby spinach leaves
lemon wedges for serving

CROQUETTES
2½ cups grated baby marrows
½ tsp crushed garlic (optional)

¼ onion, finely chopped
½ cup cake flour
1 x 170g can flaked tuna (preferably in brine), drained
salt and pepper to taste
⅓ cup crumbled feta
1 Tbsp finely chopped fresh dill
1 egg
olive oil for frying

DRESSING
1 Tbsp Greek yoghurt
1 Tbsp tangy mayonnaise
1 Tbsp olive oil
salt and pepper to taste

1. For the croquettes, combine the baby marrows, garlic (if using), onion and flour with the tuna.
2. Season with a touch of salt and pepper.
3. Add the feta, dill and egg and mix thoroughly.
4. Using your hands, roll the mixture into small balls.
5. Heat some olive oil in a pan and place the balls in the pan. Flatten them slightly with a spatula and cook for approximately 3 minutes on each side or until golden and cooked through.
6. Set aside, but keep them warm.
7. Toss the kidney beans, onion, tomatoes, yellow pepper and spinach leaves together and arrange on a platter.
8. Mix together the dressing ingredients and pour generously over the salad or serve on the side.
9. Finally, place the croquettes on top of the salad and serve with the lemon wedges on the side.

HAKE WITH *FYSTIKIA* CRUST

'*FYSTIKIA*' IS THE GREEK WORD FOR PISTACHIOS AND GREECE IS THE LARGEST EUROPEAN PRODUCER OF THESE NUTS. PISTACHIOS AREN'T JUST DELICIOUS, THEY'RE ALSO GOOD FOR YOU AS THEY ARE RICH IN POTASSIUM AND VITAMIN K. INTERESTINGLY, PISTACHIOS ARE ONE OF THE OLDEST NUTS KNOWN TO US AND ONE OF ONLY TWO NUTS MENTIONED IN THE BIBLE. THE QUEEN OF SHEBA LOVED THEM SO MUCH SHE IS SAID TO HAVE DEMANDED THAT THE ENTIRE REGION'S PISTACHIO HARVEST BE SET ASIDE FOR HER! THIS DISH GOES WELL WITH A RICE AND ROCKET ACCOMPANIMENT.

¼ cup brown and wild rice
1½ cups water
400–600g hake fillets, skinned
1 Tbsp honey
olive oil for frying
1 onion, chopped
2 cups baby spinach leaves

4 Tbsp chopped fresh dill, plus extra
for garnishing
2 cups rocket leaves
juice and grated zest of 1 lemon
salt and pepper to taste

HERB CRUST
50g shelled pistachio nuts
2 slices stale white bread,
crusts removed
1 tsp dried rosemary
1 Tbsp dried thyme
salt and pepper to taste

1. Preheat the oven to 180°C.
2. Add the rice to a saucepan and pour in the water. Bring to the boil and allow to simmer for about 20 minutes or until cooked. Drain, rinse and set aside.
3. For the herb crust, crush the pistachios in a blender.
4. Add the bread, rosemary, thyme, salt and pepper and blend again.
5. Coat the hake fillets with the honey and then cover the fish completely in the herb crust.
6. Place the fish pieces onto a greased baking tray and bake for about 6 minutes or until done.
7. In a pan, drizzle a touch of olive oil and fry the onion until translucent.
8. Add the spinach, dill and cooked rice and stir through, allowing the spinach to wilt.
9. Add the rocket leaves and mix together.
10. Squeeze the lemon juice over, add the salt and pepper and mix.
11. Finally, sprinkle the lemon zest over the rice mixture.
12. Serve immediately with the fish.

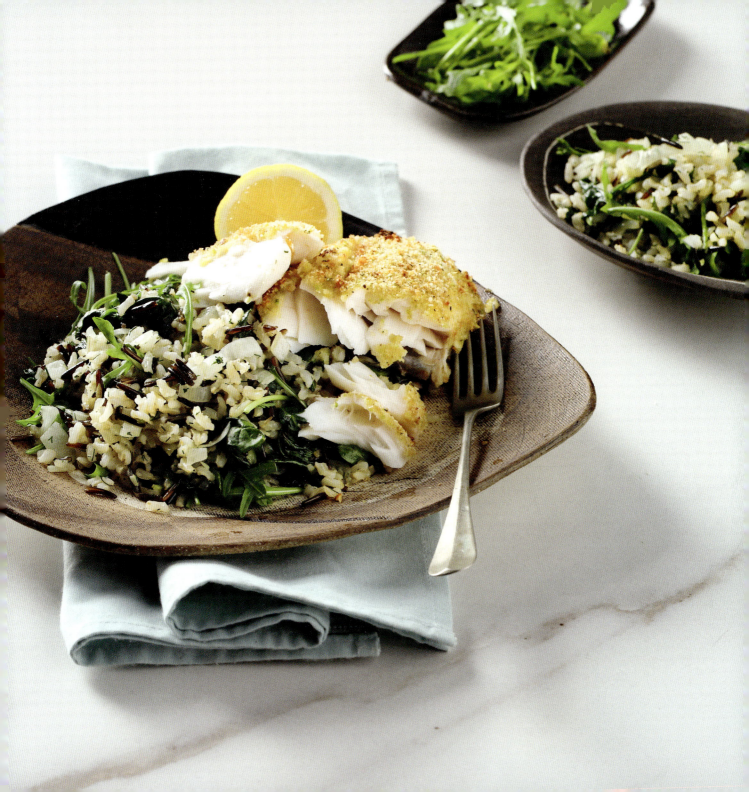

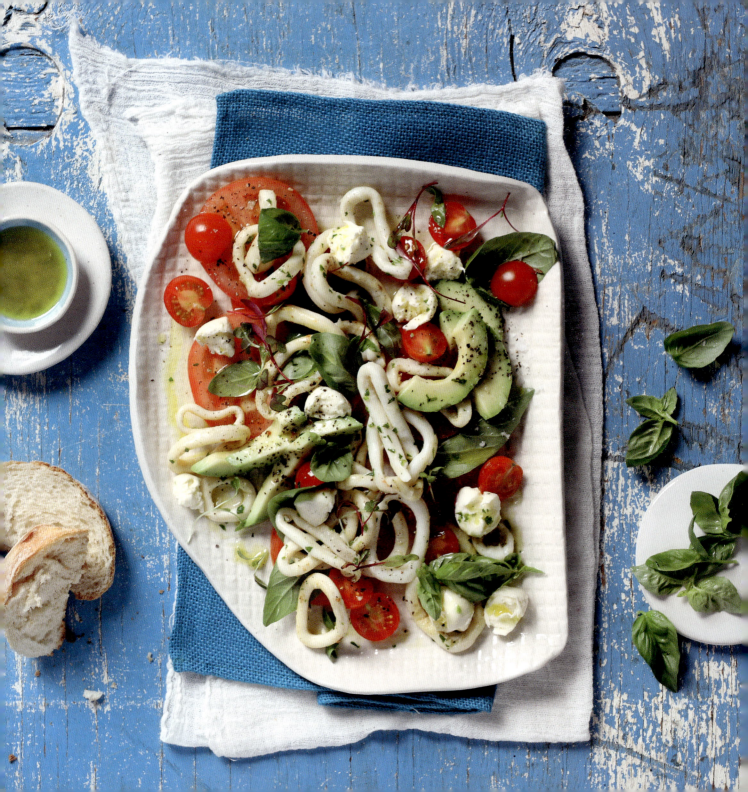

CALAMARI *CAPRESE* SALAD

CALAMARI IS READILY AVAILABLE ALONG BOTH THE MEDITERRANEAN AND SOUTH AFRICAN COASTS. TO CREATE A LIGHT MEAL, I'VE ADDED IT TO A *CAPRESE* SALAD OR *INSALATA CAPRESE*, A SALAD THAT ORIGINATED ON THE ISLAND OF CAPRI IN THE CAMPANIA REGION OF SOUTHERN ITALY. THIS COLOURFUL, VISUALLY APPEALING MEAL IS HARD TO RESIST. THE COOL, FRESH FLAVOURS ARE PERFECT FOR SERVING AT AN AL FRESCO LUNCH DURING OUR LONG, HOT SUMMERS AND I LOVE ADDING FRESH CIABATTA BREAD TO MOP UP THE EXCESS SAUCE. DO NOTE THAT THE CALAMARI NEEDS TO BE COOKED THE DAY BEFORE.

2 Tbsp olive oil

400–500g calamari rings

$\frac{1}{3}$ cup lemon juice

$\frac{1}{2}$ cup olive oil

1 clove garlic, finely chopped

1 Tbsp chopped fresh parsley

2 large tomatoes, thickly sliced

$\frac{1}{2}$ cup halved cherry tomatoes

1 x 150g tub *bocconcini* (mozzarella balls)

$\frac{1}{2}$ cup fresh basil leaves

1 avocado

salt and pepper to taste

1. In a frying pan, heat the 2 tablespoons of olive oil and fry the calamari rings, turning often, until just done (about 5 minutes). Be careful not to overcook, then leave to cool.
2. Mix the lemon juice with the half a cup of olive oil, then stir in the cooled calamari.
3. Refrigerate overnight.
4. The following day, add the garlic and parsley to the calamari mixture, stir through and allow to marinate in the fridge for at least another 2 hours.
5. To complete the rest of the dish, arrange the tomatoes and mozzarella on a platter, scatter over the basil leaves followed by the calamari rings, but reserve the marinade as a dressing.
6. Slice the avocado and arrange on top.
7. Finally, pour over the marinade dressing, season to taste and serve with fresh wholewheat rolls or ciabatta.

VALENCIA-STYLE PAELLA

VALENCIA WAS ESTABLISHED AS A COLONY BY THE ANCIENT ROMANS, WHO INTRODUCED THE CONCEPT OF IRRIGATION TO THE SETTLEMENT. CENTURIES LATER, WHEN THE MOORS WERE IN CONTROL OF SPAIN, THEY IMPROVED UPON THESE IRRIGATION SYSTEMS AND BEGAN THE CULTIVATION OF RICE AS FAR BACK AS THE 10TH CENTURY, THEREBY ESTABLISHING THE SPANISH TRADITION OF EATING RICE. THERE ARE AS MANY VERSIONS OF PAELLA AS THERE ARE INGREDIENTS. I'VE USED RISOTTO RICE, WHICH ISN'T TRADITIONAL BUT IS READILY AVAILABLE AND WORKS PERFECTLY BY ABSORBING ALL THE DELICIOUS FLAVOURS. SMOKED PAPRIKA, OR PIMENTO AS IT'S KNOWN IN SPAIN, ADDS A WONDERFUL SMOKINESS TO ANY DISH AND IS A STAPLE IN EVERY SPANISH KITCHEN.

---

a pinch of saffron

2 Tbsp white wine

olive oil for frying

110g chorizo, sliced

400g prawns, shelled and deveined

½ tsp minced chilli

2 lemons, plus extra for serving

1 onion, chopped

1 clove garlic, finely chopped

3–4 chicken breast fillets, cut into large chunks

1 cup uncooked risotto rice

4 heaped tsp tomato paste

4 artichoke hearts, chopped

2 tsp smoked paprika

2 cups chicken stock

1 cup frozen peas

4 cooked prawns for garnishing, head and tail still intact

salt and pepper to taste

fresh parsley for garnishing

1. Soak the saffron threads in the white wine for about 10 minutes.
2. Heat a touch of olive oil in a cast-iron pan and fry the chorizo until crispy. Remove and set aside.
3. To the same pan, add the prawns, chilli and juice of a quarter of a lemon, then fry until the prawns just turn pink. Remove with a slotted spoon and set aside.
4. Add the onion and garlic to the pan and cook until the onion has softened, but not browned.
5. Add the chicken pieces and fry until browned.
6. Return the chorizo to the pan, along with the rice. Mix well, toasting the rice for about 3 minutes.
7. Add the saffron and wine, tomato paste, artichokes, paprika and chicken stock.
8. Cover, bring rapidly to the boil and boil for about 10 minutes.
9. When most of the liquid has been absorbed, return the prawns to the pan and add the peas.
10. Cook for another few minutes then remove from the heat but keep covered and leave to rest for another 5 minutes.
11. Squeeze the balance of the lemons over all.
12. Arrange the intact cooked prawns on top, season to taste, garnish with the parsley and serve immediately with extra lemon wedges on the side.

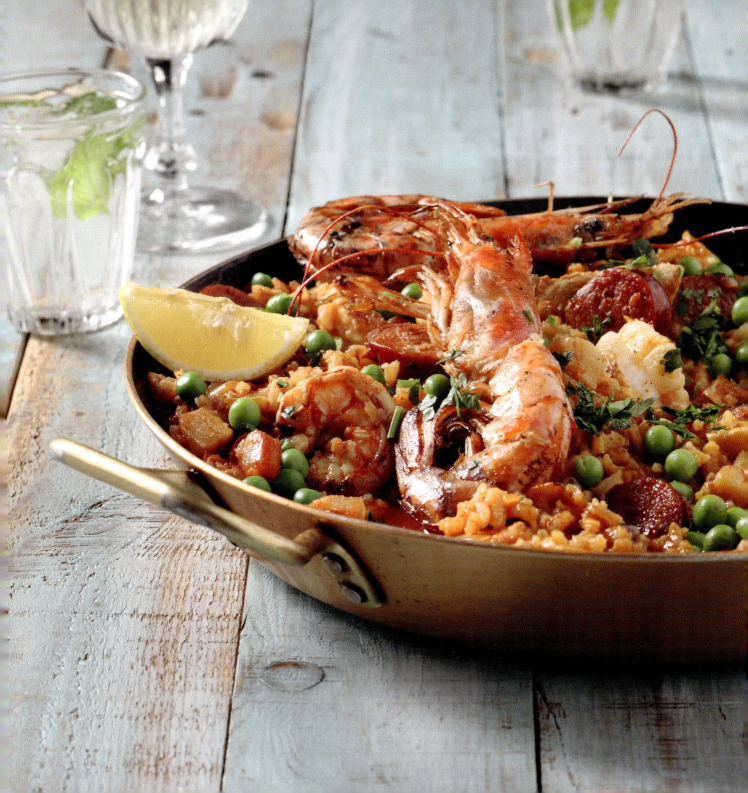

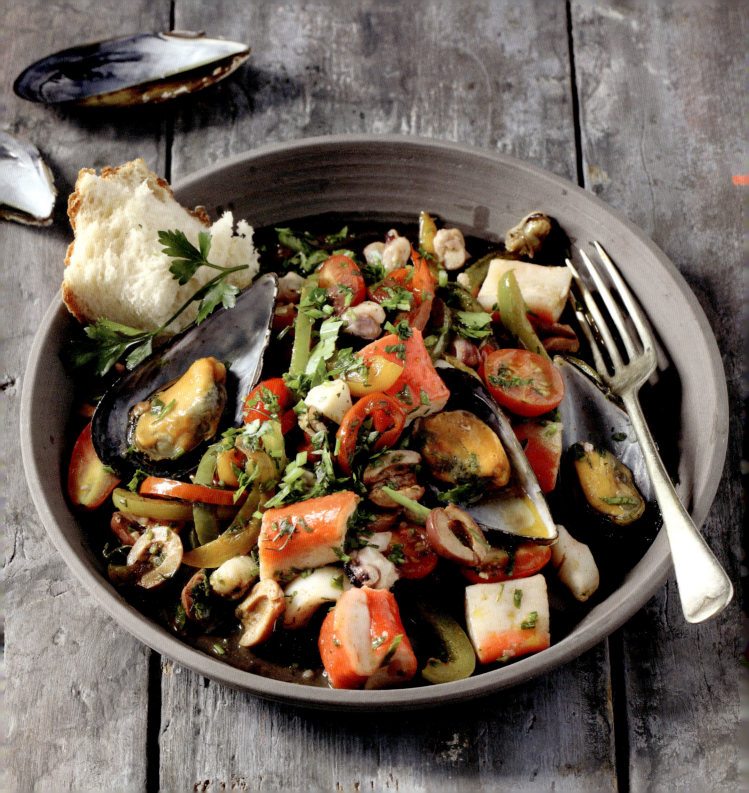

ENSALADA DE MARISCOS (SEAFOOD SALAD)

SEAFOOD IS ABUNDANT ALONG THE COAST OF SPAIN AND WE ARE LUCKY ENOUGH TO BE BLESSED WITH GOOD STOCKS IN SOUTH AFRICA AS WELL. READY-MIXED SEAFOOD IS AVAILABLE IN MOST SUPERMARKETS AND CREATES A FRESH COMBINATION OF TASTES AND TEXTURES THAT IS VISUALLY ATTRACTIVE AND DELICIOUS TO EAT. THIS REFRESHING SUMMER SALAD IS JUST WHAT YOU NEED WHEN THE SUN IS BLAZING OUTSIDE.

800g seafood mix: prawns, mussels, calamari, crabsticks
juice of 1 lemon
salt and pepper to taste
1 Tbsp olive oil
½ green pepper, sliced into strips
½ red pepper, sliced into strips
½ yellow pepper, sliced into strips
16 pitted black olives, halved
½ tsp smoked paprika

16 rosa tomatoes, halved
2 Tbsp chopped fresh parsley
2 Tbsp chopped fresh dill

DRESSING
¼ cup olive oil
2 Tbsp sherry vinegar
½ tsp mustard powder (your choice of strength)
salt and pepper to taste

1. Steam the seafood mix until just cooked.
2. Remove from the heat, drizzle the lemon juice over the mix, stir to coat and leave to cool.
3. Heat the olive oil in a non-stick pan and gently sauté the peppers, olives and smoked paprika until the peppers soften slightly. Set aside to cool.
4. Stir the tomatoes into the cooled seafood mix, along with the peppers and olives.
5. Add the parsley and dill and stir through.
6. Whisk the dressing ingredients together and pour over the entire salad. Toss to coat well.
7. Serve chilled with some bread to soak up the dressing.

BODRUM FISH SALAD

TURKEY IS FAMOUS FOR ITS SPICES AND A VISIT TO ISTANBUL'S SPICE BAZAAR WILL SHOW YOU WHY. ROWS OF FRESHLY GROUND SPICES LINE THE ALLEYWAYS AND AISLES OF THIS HISTORIC MARKET. BUT YOU DON'T HAVE TO GO TO ISTANBUL TO ENJOY THE FLAVOURS. SUMAC IS AVAILABLE IN OUR STORES; IT'S A VERSATILE SPICE WITH A TANGY, LEMONY FLAVOUR, PERFECT FOR FISH. IN THIS RECIPE, SUMAC ADDS COLOUR AND SPICINESS, MINT THE FRESHNESS AND FETA A SILKY FINISH. BODRUM WAS ORIGINALLY A LITTLE TURKISH FISHING VILLAGE WHERE THE LOCALS CHOSE THEIR FISH, STRAIGHT OFF THE FISHING BOATS.

2–3 baby brinjals or 1 large brinjal, sliced into rounds
olive oil for frying
500– 600g yellowtail fillets (or any other firm white fish)
2–4 Tbsp ground sumac
salt and pepper to taste
1 x 410g can lentils, drained
4 stalks celery, sliced
4 spring onions, sliced

¼ cup crumbled feta
1 Tbsp chopped fresh mint
1 Tbsp chopped fresh parsley
4–6 Peppadews, sliced
¼ cup lemon juice
½ tsp prepared Dijon mustard
¼ cup olive oil
4–8 cos lettuce leaves, depending on size
chopped fresh parsley for garnishing

1. Sauté the brinjal slices in a little oil, until cooked. Set aside on absorbent kitchen towel.
2. Cut the fish into large chunks and season liberally with the sumac.
3. Heat a pan with a little oil and fry the fish, turning occasionally, until cooked. Set aside, but keep warm and season with salt and pepper.
4. Mix together the lentils, celery, spring onions, feta, mint, parsley and Peppadews.
5. Blend together the lemon juice, mustard, salt and pepper, and a quarter cup of olive oil. Pour over the lentil mixture and stir to ensure that the ingredients are well coated.
6. Separate the lettuce leaves and arrange individual leaves on each plate. Spoon in the lentil mixture.
7. Place the brinjal slices next to the lettuce leaves and arrange a portion of fish on top.
8. Garnish with the parsley. Serve with wedges of lemon, if you like.

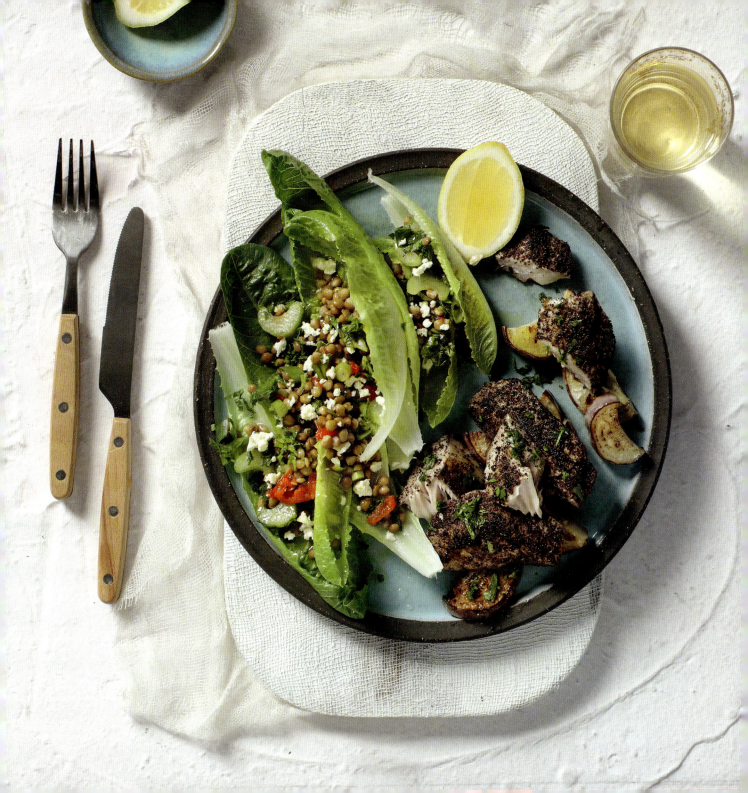

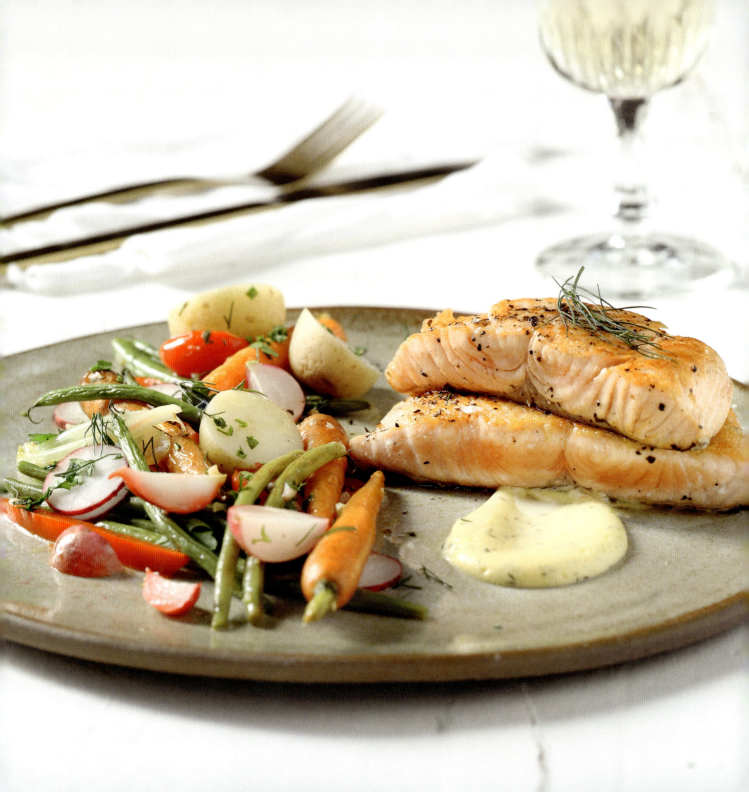

SALMON WITH VEGETABLES PROVENÇAL

THIS DELECTABLE BLEND OF TEXTURES, COLOURS AND FLAVOURS IS REMINISCENT OF THE VIBRANT FOOD MARKETS OF PROVENCE, WHICH BORDERS THE MEDITERRANEAN ALONG THE SOUTHEASTERN COAST OF FRANCE.

8 baby carrots, with their tops
6 Tbsp olive oil
4 radishes, quartered
24 extra fine green beans
1 red pepper, sliced into strips
½ onion, finely chopped
¾ tsp minced garlic

8 rosa tomatoes, halved
400–500g salmon fillets
salt and pepper to taste
12 baby potatoes

LEMON SAUCE
½ cup freshly squeezed lemon juice

(from ± 2 lemons, retain the lemons)
2 egg yolks
3 Tbsp water
2 Tbsp chopped fresh dill
salt
2 Tbsp Greek yoghurt

1. Preheat the oven to 190°C.
2. Coat the carrots in 1 tablespoon of the olive oil, transfer into an ovenproof dish and roast for about 5 minutes.
3. Add the radishes, green beans, red pepper, onion and garlic to the carrots, along with another 2 tablespoons of olive oil. Mix well to ensure that all the vegetables are coated with the oil and garlic.
4. Add the juiced lemons (for extra flavour, but remove before serving). Roast for 10 minutes, then add the tomatoes and roast for another 10 minutes.
5. Season the salmon fillets with salt and pepper.
6. Heat a non-stick pan until hot, add the fillets and cook for about 3 minutes per side, or until the salmon is cooked but still pink in the middle. Set aside and keep warm.
7. For the sauce, pour the lemon juice into a saucepan, add the egg yolks and whisk. Add the water and continue whisking over a low heat until the mixture starts to thicken, but remove from heat if the eggs begin to 'scramble'.
8. Add the dill and season with salt.
9. Add the yoghurt and whisk well. Remove from the heat once the sauce is heated through and thickened.
10. Cook the baby potatoes in boiling water until done.
11. To serve, arrange the mixed vegetables on each plate, place a salmon fillet on top and the potatoes to the side. Serve the lemon sauce on the side, garnish as desired and serve immediately.

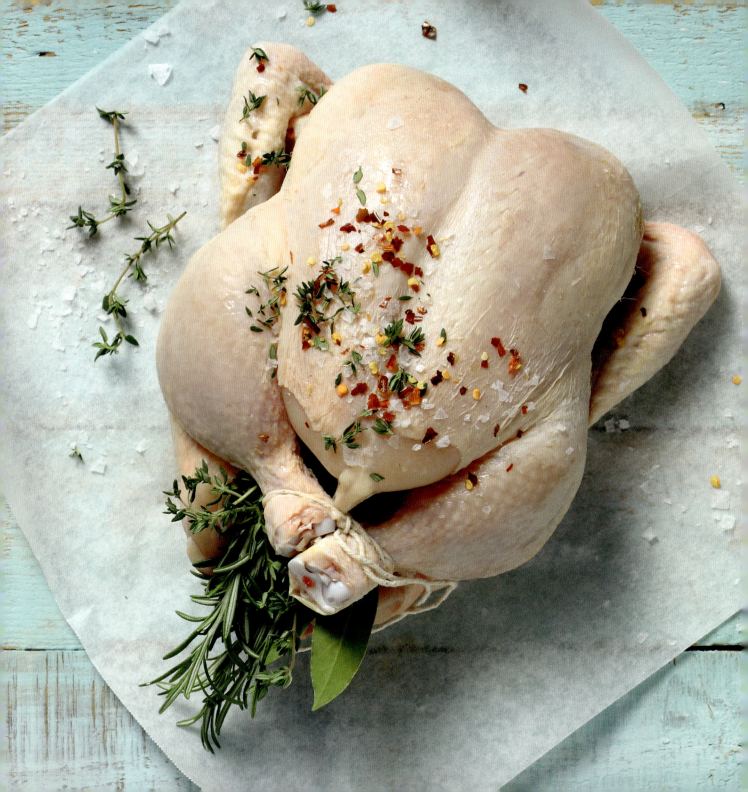

CHICKEN

Chicken served in the Mediterranean region is invariably free range and always incorporates plenty of additional flavours, herbs and spices. It is such a versatile white meat and may be served hot or cold. Chicken is low in fat, high in protein and rich in minerals such as phosphorous and calcium. What's more, it contains two nutrients that are good for relieving stress, tryptophan and vitamin B5 – both of which have a calming effect on the body.

Poultry is immensely popular and is often cooked simply by roasting or sautéing so that the taste and quality of the meat may be fully appreciated. The people along the Mediterranean eat a wide range of game poultry, including guinea fowl, partridge and quail. Although game poultry is not as popular in South Africa, if you're feeling adventurous feel free to substitute one of these options for chicken, but remember to change your cooking time accordingly.

Though prices have risen in recent years, chicken remains an affordable white meat. You may pay a premium for free range, but you will usually find the additional investment is worth it as the meat is generally more flavourful and satisfying.

Chicken is generally easy to prepare and the perfect partner to so many ingredients. Whether you're tucking into the traditional Chicken Cacciatore or having an elegant dinner with chicken parcels, you'll find something suitable for every occasion.

CHICKEN *LEMNOS*

LEMONS ARE A STAPLE OF MANY GREEK DISHES AND THE LEMON IS CERTAINLY THE STAR INGREDIENT HERE. BY STUFFING THE CHICKEN CAVITY WITH LEMONS AND HERBS YOU'RE LITERALLY INFUSING THE CHICKEN FROM THE INSIDE OUT. IT IS THOUGHT LEMONS ORIGINATED IN INDIA, BUT THEY WERE ALSO KNOWN TO THE ANCIENT ROMANS. THEY BECAME MORE COMMON IN EUROPE AROUND THE 12TH CENTURY. THESE VERSATILE FRUITS ALSO OFFER MANY HEALTH BENEFITS AND HAVE A DETOXIFYING AND CLEANSING EFFECT ON THE BODY.

1.2kg whole free-range chicken
salt and pepper to taste
½ Tbsp dried thyme
2 lemons, quartered
4 cloves garlic, halved

1 Tbsp olive oil
1 onion, sliced into wedges
½ cup water
½ cup chicken stock
5–6 sprigs of fresh thyme

1. Preheat the oven to 180°C.
2. Season the chicken cavity with salt, pepper and half of the dried thyme.
3. Stuff 5 of the lemon quarters into the chicken cavity, along with half of the garlic cloves.
4. Place the chicken in a roasting dish.
5. Drizzle the olive oil over the bird and rub well into the skin, followed by the balance of the thyme.
6. Arrange the onion wedges around the chicken, along with the remaining garlic.
7. Pour in the water and chicken stock.
8. Cover and roast in the oven for 30 minutes.
9. Remove the lid, sprinkle over the fresh thyme and continue roasting for another hour.
10. Remove the chicken from the roasting dish, cover and leave to rest for at least 10 minutes before serving.
11. Use the cooking juices as gravy.
12. Serve the onions with the chicken, as well as the remaining lemon wedges. A salad with brinjals, tomatoes and cucumber (see page35) will make a perfect accompaniment to this dish.

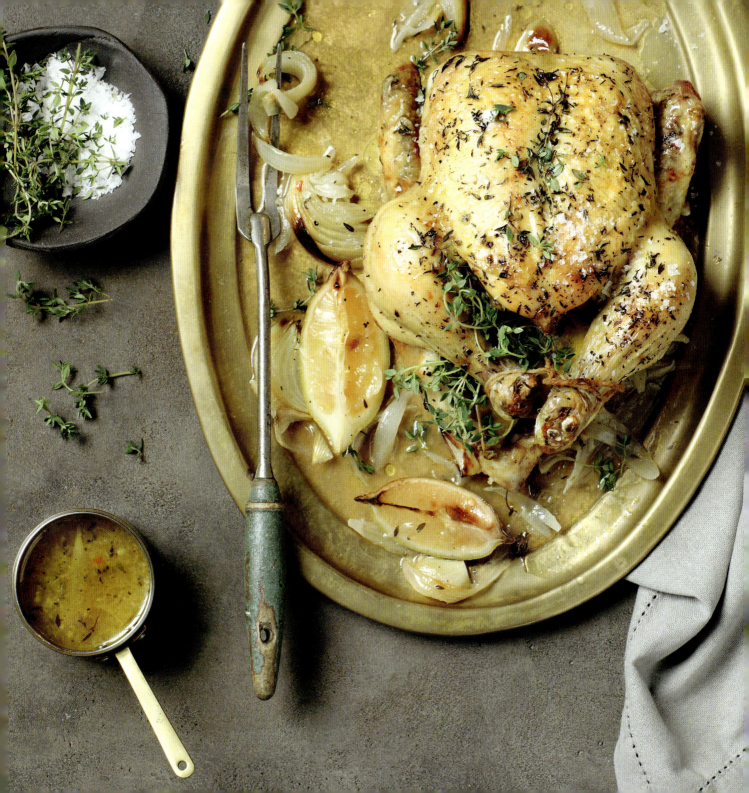

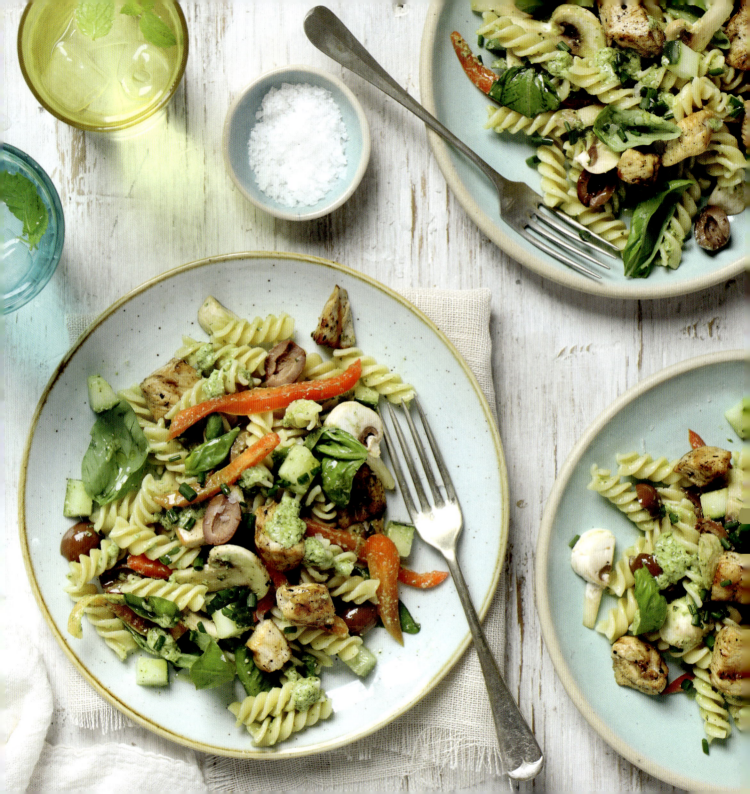

PASTA *POLLO*

PASTA IS OFTEN SEEN AS AN UNHEALTHY INGREDIENT, BUT MORE OFTEN THAN NOT IT'S THE RICH, CREAMY, CHEESY SAUCE THAT PACKS ON THE CALORIES, AND NOT THE PASTA. FUSILLI IS A GOOD PASTA FOR THIS DISH AS THE SAUCE BECOMES TRAPPED IN THE SPIRALS. THE YOGHURT AND PESTO CREATE THE CREAM, THE CUCUMBER ADDS THE CRUNCH, OLIVES THE TARTNESS AND THE CHICKEN PROVIDES THE PROTEIN, ALL IN ONE HEALTHY DISH FILLED WITH THE FRESH FLAVOURS OF ITALY. '*POLLO*' MEANS CHICKEN IN ITALIAN (AND SPANISH).

4–6 chicken breast fillets, cubed small
200–300g fusilli
1 cup chopped mushrooms
½ cup sliced black olives
1 red pepper, sliced into strips
½ cup chopped cucumber
2 Tbsp chopped fresh basil
chopped fresh chives for garnishing

DRESSING
¼ cup basil pesto
3 Tbsp Greek yoghurt
¼ cup olive oil
salt and pepper to taste

1. In a preheated griddle pan, sauté the chicken until just cooked. Add a touch of water if necessary. Set aside.
2. Cook the pasta according to the packet instructions until *al dente*. Drain and leave to cool.
3. In a serving bowl, combine the cooled pasta with the mushrooms, olives, red pepper, cucumber and basil.
4. Spoon in the chicken and toss.
5. Blend the dressing ingredients together until smooth.
6. Pour over the pasta and toss well or serve on the side, if you prefer.
7. Garnish with the chives before serving.

CANNES CHICKEN PHYLLO PARCELS

THIS DISH REQUIRES A LITTLE WORK, BUT IT'S DEFINITELY WORTH IT. THE DELICIOUS LITTLE PARCELS LOOK LIKE THE WORK OF A SERIOUS CHEF AT A SWISH RESTAURANT ALONG THE CÔTE D'AZUR. PREPARE FOR A SURPRISE IN YOUR MOUTH WHEN YOU FIRST EXPERIENCE THE CREAMINESS OF THE SAUCE ACCOMPANIED BY THE PIQUANCY OF THE PEPPADEWS. PERFECT WITH AN ICE-CHILLED ROSÉ.

4 chicken breast fillets
salt and pepper to taste
olive oil for frying
4–5 white button mushrooms, finely chopped
½ onion, finely chopped
½ tsp minced garlic
½ tsp dried mixed herbs
± 3 sheets phyllo pastry

2 Tbsp melted butter
± 1 cup baby spinach leaves
8–10 slices mozzarella
3–4 baby marrows, sliced lengthways
4–5 mild Peppadews, quartered
± 1 Tbsp sesame seeds
2 tsp chopped chives for garnishing

MUSTARD CREAM DRESSING
150g Greek yoghurt
1 heaped tsp prepared wholegrain mustard
salt and pepper to taste

1. Preheat the oven to 180°C.
2. Flatten the chicken breasts with a mallet and, if they are large, cut in half before seasoning with salt and pepper.
3. In a frying pan, fry the breasts in a little olive oil until browned and just cooked through. Place on absorbent kitchen paper and set aside.
4. Add the mushrooms, onion, salt, pepper, garlic and mixed herbs to the same frying pan and fry in a little oil until softened. Remove and set aside.
5. Cut the phyllo sheets in half, lengthways, and brush each with melted butter. Towards one end of each sheet, place a few spinach leaves – about the size of the chicken breast – followed by a teaspoonful of the mushroom mixture.
6. Place a chicken breast on top of the mushroom mixture and follow this with layers of the mozzarella (about 2 slices per breast), baby marrows and Peppadews. Finally, cover the stack with more spinach leaves.
7. Wrap the phyllo sheet around the layers, as you would wrap a gift. Brush the whole phyllo parcel with melted butter, plus extra over the folded ends so that they stick together. Sprinkle the sesame seeds over the tops.
8. Place the parcels on a non-stick baking tray and bake in the oven until browned (5–10 minutes).
9. To make the dressing, heat the ingredients together.
10. Arrange the chicken parcels on a serving platter, pour over the warm dressing and scatter the chives on top.
11. Serve immediately, preferably with Grilled Asparagus (see page 75).

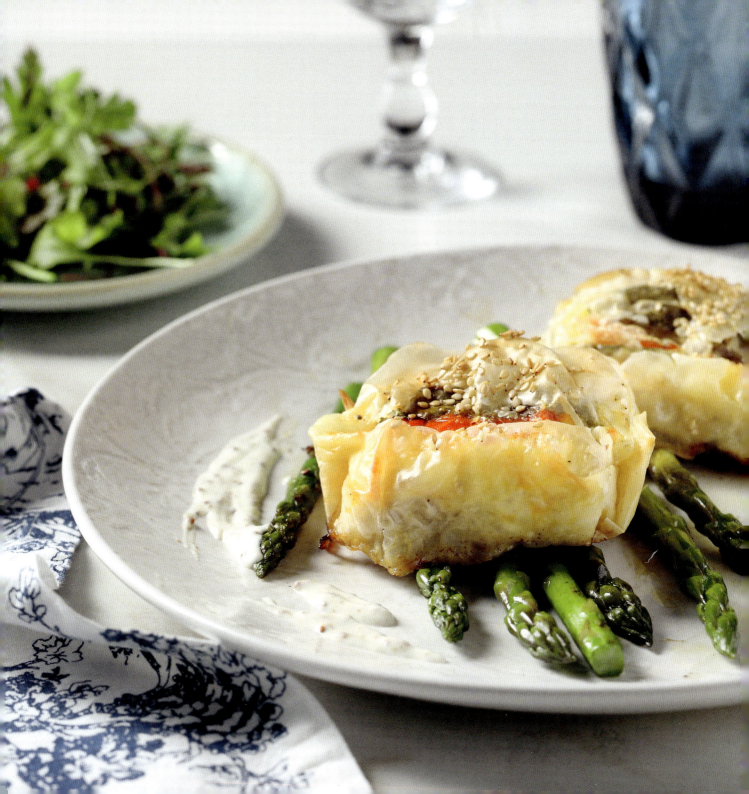

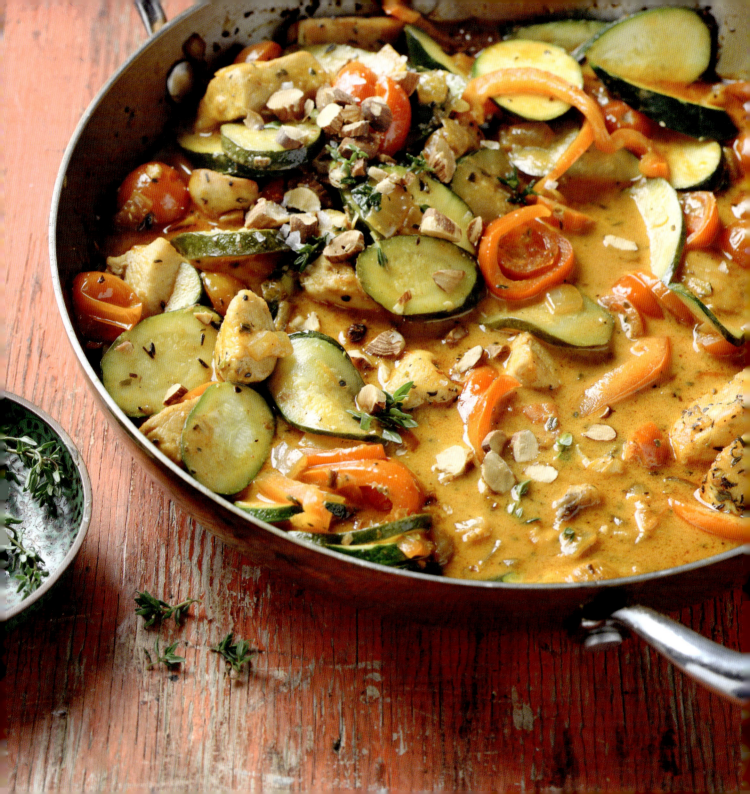

CHICKEN RAMBLAS

THERE IS A STREET IN BARCELONA CALLED THE RAMBLAS, WHERE YOU CAN FIND A BIT OF EVERYTHING, FROM FLOWER SELLERS AND ARTISTS TO ASTOUNDING FOOD MARKETS SERVING A POTPOURRI OF SPANISH FLAVOURS. THIS DISH IS A BIT LIKE THAT. IT'S PERFECT FOR USING UP LEFTOVERS, SO FEEL FREE TO SUBSTITUTE AS MUCH AS YOU LIKE. GENEROUS AMOUNTS OF DIFFERENT VEGETABLES WILL PROVIDE YOU WITH YOUR DAILY DOSE OF MINERALS AND NUTRIENTS. HOT PEPPADEWS ARE THE EQUIVALENT OF HOT PEPPER FLAKES, WHICH, ALONG WITH PAPRIKA AND ALMONDS, ARE TYPICAL OF SPANISH CUISINE.

3–4 chicken breast fillets

2 Tbsp dried thyme

salt and pepper to taste

2 Tbsp olive oil

1 onion, chopped

½ tsp minced garlic

1 red pepper, sliced into strips

4 tsp paprika

4 tsp dried origanum

8–10 baby marrows, sliced on the diagonal

10–15 cherry tomatoes, halved

¾ cup tropical fruit juice

8 tsp medium fat yoghurt

1½ cups cooked brown rice

4 hot Peppadews, chopped

roasted chopped almonds for garnishing

1. Slice the chicken fillets in half lengthways, then chop into cubes.
2. Season with thyme, salt and pepper.
3. Add the olive oil to a pan and sauté the chicken until browned and just cooked. Remove the chicken from the pan and keep warm.
4. In the same pan, gently fry the onion in a touch of oil, until softened.
5. Add the garlic and fry for another minute.
6. Stir in the red pepper, paprika and origanum. Cook for a few minutes, stirring often.
7. Add the baby marrows and tomatoes and stir through.
8. Pour in the juice, add the chicken pieces and stir. Leave to simmer for a few minutes.
9. Season to taste.
10. Gradually stir in the yoghurt.
11. Spoon about a quarter cup of rice onto each plate and add the Peppadews on top.
12. Add some of the chicken mixture to the rest of the plate, sprinkle over the roasted almonds, garnish as desired and serve immediately.

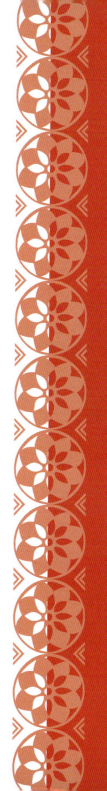

CHICKEN VÉRONIQUE

'VÉRONIQUE' IS OFTEN THE NAME GIVEN TO FRENCH DISHES THAT FEATURE SEEDLESS WHITE GRAPES. THE TERM WAS COINED IN 1907 BY THE FATHER OF MODERN CUISINE, AUGUSTE ESCOFFIER, IN HONOUR OF A COMIC OPERA. THE SWEET GRAPES, RICH IN VITAMINS C AND K, BALANCE PERFECTLY WITH THE SALTY BACON. BOTH INFUSE THE CHICKEN WITH EXTRA FLAVOUR. BACON IS ONE OF THE OLDEST PROCESSED MEATS IN THE WORLD. IT'S BELIEVED THE CHINESE WERE ALREADY SALTING PORK 3 500 YEARS AGO.

4 chicken breast fillets

salt and pepper to taste

2 lemons, sliced

1 x 200g packet bacon

½ onion, sliced

1 cup dessert wine or sherry

½ cup chicken stock

½ cup white grapes

4 Tbsp Greek yoghurt

fresh chives for garnishing

1. Preheat the oven to 180°C.
2. Flatten the chicken fillets with a mallet, then season with salt and pepper.
3. Place slices of lemon on top of each fillet, then wrap the fillets with bacon (about 2 rashers per fillet).
4. Arrange in an ovenproof dish and scatter over the onion slices.
5. Pour over half of the wine or sherry and bake, uncovered, for 30 minutes.
6. In the meanwhile, heat the chicken stock in a pot and add the rest of the wine. Leave to simmer until reduced by half.
7. When the chicken is ready, remove it from the oven but keep warm.
8. Pour the remainder of the chicken cooking liquid, along with the onions, into the chicken and wine sauce and stir.
9. Add the grapes and leave to simmer for about 5 minutes or until the grapes are heated through.
10. Stir in the yoghurt or serve on the side.
11. Pour the sauce over the chicken, garnish with the chives and serve immediately.
12. This dish is best served with Green Beans and Mushrooms (see page 68).

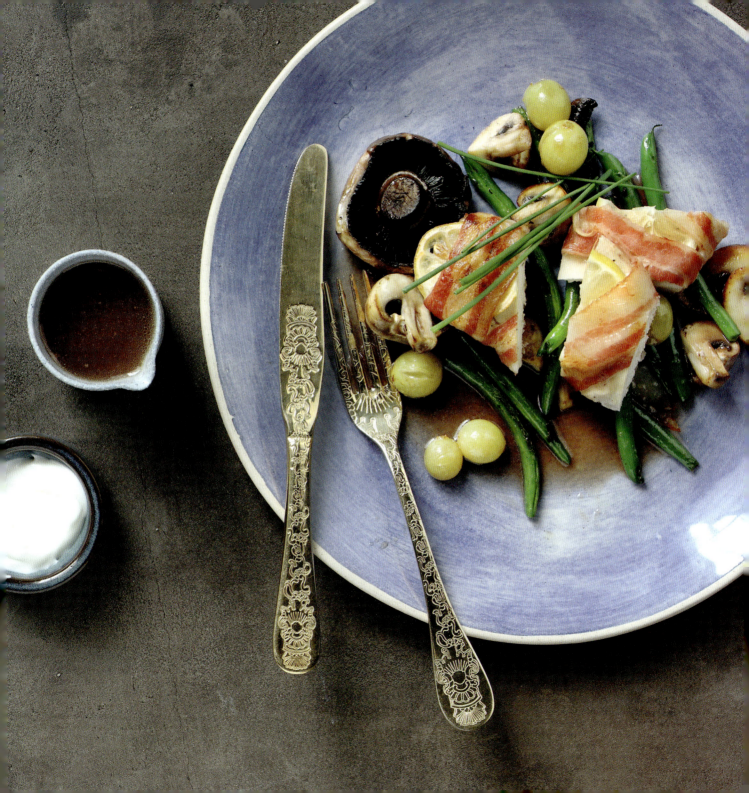

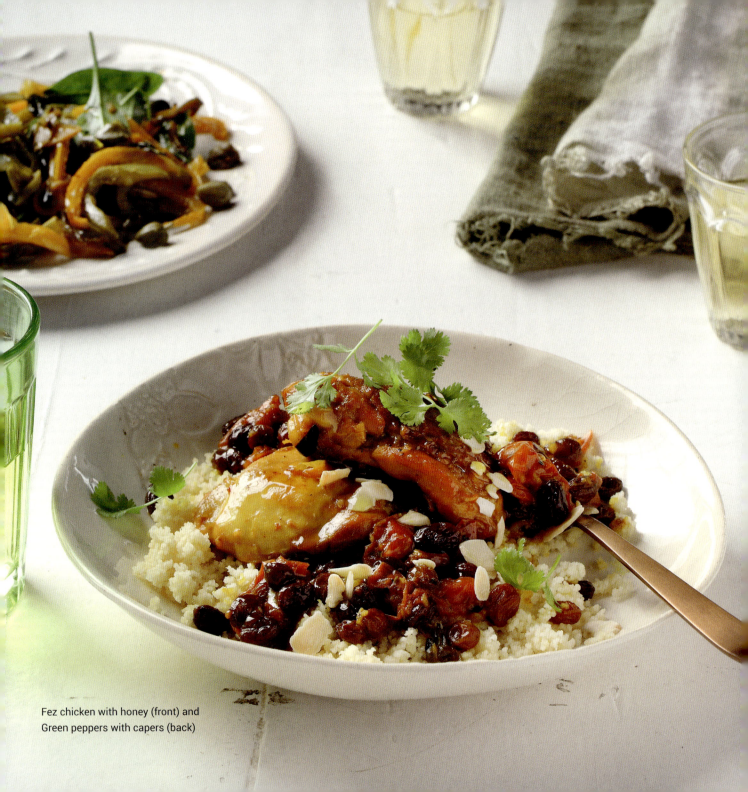

Fez chicken with honey (front) and
Green peppers with capers (back)

FEZ CHICKEN WITH HONEY

TURMERIC'S DISTINCTIVE SHADE OF ORANGE IS DERIVED FROM ITS HIGH CURCUMIN CONTENT. IT IS ONE OF THE MOST FREQUENTLY MENTIONED MEDICINAL PLANTS IN THE WORLD. ARGUABLY, MORE STUDIES HAVE BEEN CONDUCTED ON ITS BENEFITS THAN ON ANY OTHER HERB OR SPICE, DUE TO ITS POWERFUL ANTI-INFLAMMATORY AND HEALING PROPERTIES, COMPARABLE TO – AND PERHAPS EVEN BETTER THAN – OVER-THE-COUNTER MEDICINES. COMMONLY USED IN MOROCCAN COOKING, HERE IT IS JUXTAPOSED WITH DELICATE HONEY TO CREATE A PERFECT BALANCE OF FLAVOURS.

8–10 chicken thighs

¼ cup olive oil

1 piece stick cinnamon

4 cups chicken stock

12 cherry tomatoes, halved

salt and pepper to taste

½ tsp turmeric

2 Tbsp minced ginger

¼ cup honey

½ cup seedless raisins

¼ cup flaked almonds

fresh parsley for garnishing

1. In a saucepan, brown the chicken pieces in the olive oil, then add the cinnamon, chicken stock, tomatoes, salt and pepper.
2. Bring to the boil and leave to simmer for about 35 minutes.
3. Add the turmeric, ginger, honey and raisins and leave to simmer for another 10 minutes, allowing the liquid to reduce by two-thirds.
4. Garnish with the almonds and parsley.
5. Best served with couscous and Green Peppers with Capers (see page 74).

SEVILLE CHICKEN SALAD

SEVILLE IS FAMOUS FOR ITS GOTHIC LANDSCAPE, AS WELL AS ITS ORANGES. THE HEADY SCENT OF ORANGE BLOSSOM IS A PURE DELIGHT, CREATING A FRAGRANT AND ROMANTIC SPRING ATMOSPHERE. SEVILLE MARMALADE CAN BE ENJOYED ALL YEAR ROUND AND ISN'T ONLY GOOD ON TOAST. SMEARED OVER CHICKEN, IT CREATES A TASTE EXPLOSION ON THE PALATE. BY POACHING THE CHICKEN IN ORANGE JUICE, IT NOT ONLY ENHANCES THE ORANGE FLAVOUR BUT SOFTENS THE CHICKEN TO CREATE A SUCCULENT, TASTY DISH THAT CONTRASTS WELL WITH THE TANGY CABBAGE AND OLIVES.

4–5 chicken breast fillets, cut into strips

1 tsp dried thyme

salt and pepper to taste

1 Tbsp orange marmalade

olive oil for frying

½ cup white wine

½ cup orange juice

¼ cup water or chicken stock

1 yellow pepper, sliced into strips

1½ cups shredded red cabbage

1½ cups shredded green cabbage

1½ cups baby spinach leaves

1 cup pitted black olives

micro greens for garnishing

orange wedges for serving

DRESSING

¼ cup olive oil

2 Tbsp orange juice

salt and pepper to taste

1. Season the chicken strips with the thyme, salt and pepper.
2. Coat the strips with the marmalade.
3. Pour the olive oil into a pan and brown the chicken pieces.
4. Pour in the wine and orange juice and poach the chicken until cooked through. If it becomes too dry, add a little chicken stock or orange juice to moisten the chicken.
5. Once cooked through, set aside.
6. On a platter, combine the yellow pepper, both types of cabbage, spinach and olives.
7. Mix the dressing ingredients together, pour over the salad then arrange the chicken slices on top.
8. Garnish with the micro greens and serve with orange wedges.

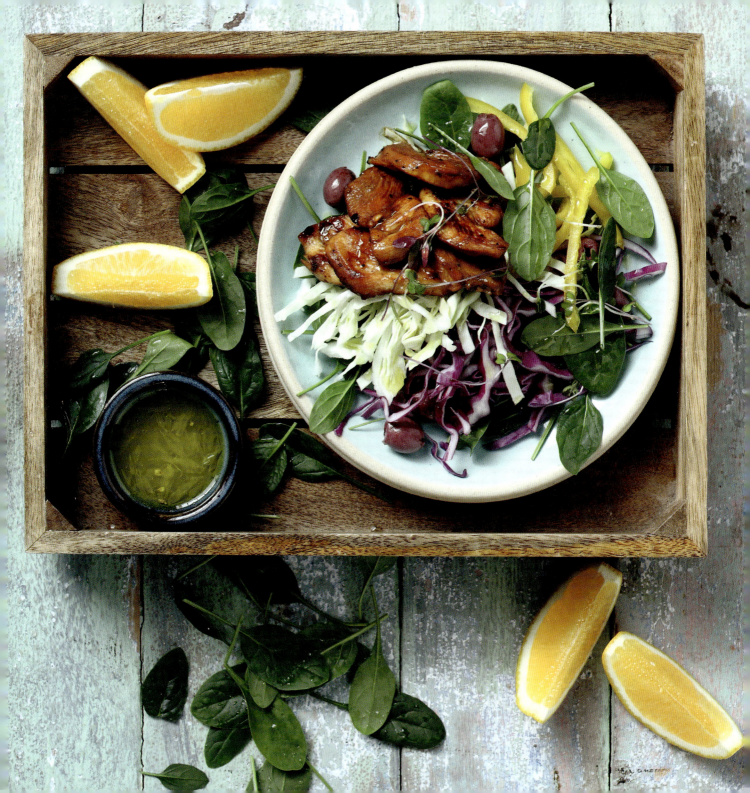

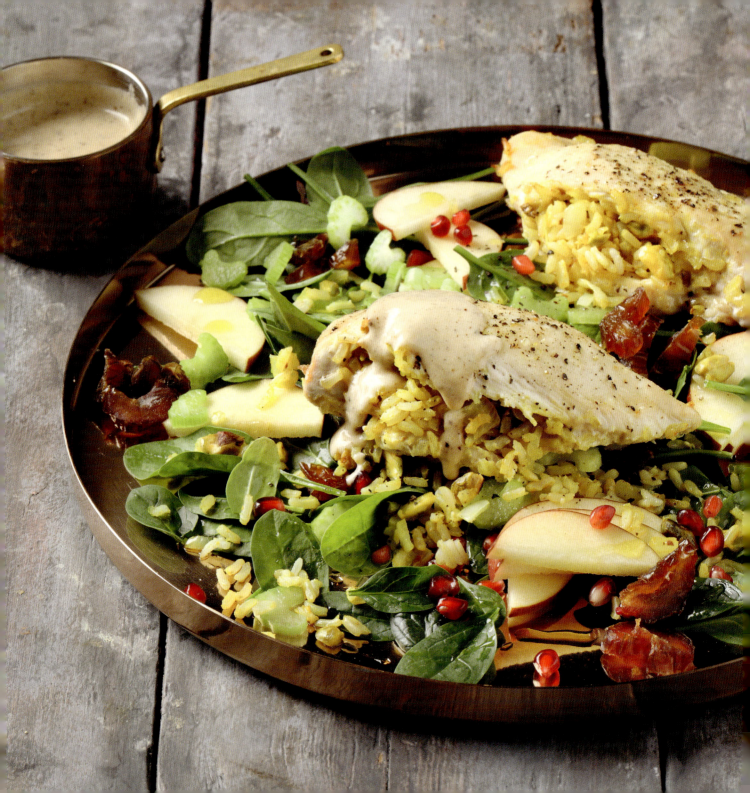

MOREISH MOROCCAN CHICKEN SALAD

MOROCCO IS FAMOUS FOR ITS RICH SPICES AND FLAVOURFUL FOOD, AND THIS DISH IS A MIXTURE OF THESE TASTE SENSATIONS. THE CARDAMOM PROVIDES THE AROMA, TURMERIC THE COLOUR AND THE PISTACHIOS THE CRUNCH. THE CHICKEN'S FLAVOUR BALANCES PERFECTLY WITH THE SWEET, CHEWY DATES AND TART APPLES, WHILE THE POMEGRANATE PROVIDES THE FINISHING TOUCH.

olive oil for frying
½ onion, chopped
½ tsp crushed garlic
20 pistachio nuts, shelled and
  roughly chopped
2 Tbsp roughly chopped pine nuts
1 cup cooked brown rice
seeds of 2 cardamon pods
½ tsp turmeric

salt and pepper to taste
4–6 chicken breast fillets
¼ cup white wine vinegar
1 unpeeled red apple, chopped
3 stalks celery, chopped
2 pitted dates, chopped
2 cups baby spinach leaves
2 Tbsp pomegranate arils

SAUCE
1 tsp sumac powder
100ml chicken stock
juice of ½ lemon
½ cup plain yoghurt
½ tsp grated nutmeg
salt and pepper to taste

1. Preheat the oven to 180°C.
2. In a pan, heat a little olive oil and sauté the onion and garlic until the onion is translucent.
3. Add all the nuts and rice to the onion and garlic mixture and sauté for another minute or so.
4. Stir in the cardamom seeds, turmeric, salt and pepper, then sauté for about 3 minutes. Remove from the heat.
5. Cut pockets lengthways into the chicken breasts and stuff with the rice mixture.
6. Place the chicken breasts in an ovenproof dish, drizzle generously with olive oil and pour 1 tablespoon of the vinegar over each chicken breast. Season generously with salt and pepper.
7. Cover with a lid or aluminium foil and bake for approximately 20 minutes.
8. Remove the lid or foil and grill for another 5 minutes to brown the tops of the breasts.
9. For the sauce, add the sumac, chicken stock and lemon juice to a pan and simmer until reduced by a third. Add the yoghurt and nutmeg. Season with salt and pepper and stir occasionally, until the sauce begins to thicken.
10. Combine the apple, celery and dates.
11. Arrange the spinach leaves on a platter and place the apple and celery mixture over the leaves. Season with salt and pepper. Scatter over any leftover rice mixture.
12. Place the chicken breasts on top of the salad ingredients and pour over the sauce.
13. Sprinkle the pomegranate arils over all.

TURKISH KEBABS

TURKEY IS FAMOUS FOR ITS KEBABS, TRADITIONALLY COOKED OVER OPEN COALS. ANOTHER TURKISH TRADITION IS TO MARINATE MEAT IN YOGHURT. MARINADE ADDS FLAVOUR AND MOISTURE TO A DISH, AND DAIRY-BASED MARINADES TRULY TENDERISE MEAT BECAUSE THEY'RE ONLY MILDLY ACIDIC. THIS MEANS THEY DON'T TOUGHEN THE MEAT LIKE SOME STRONGER, ACIDIC MARINADES TEND TO DO. THE ADDITION OF CUMIN AND CAYENNE PEPPER TO THE YOGHURT ENSURES THAT THE TRULY AUTHENTIC FLAVOURS OF TURKEY DEVELOP IN THE MEAT. THE CREAMY *CACIK* AND TOMATO SALAD ROUND OFF THIS SUPERB MEAL WITH ITS SUBTLE EVOCATION OF OTTOMAN TRADITIONS.

4–6 chicken breast fillets
½ cup Greek yoghurt
¼ cup olive oil
2 Tbsp red wine vinegar
1 x 50g sachet tomato paste
1 tsp crushed garlic

2 tsp ground cumin
½ tsp cayenne pepper
juice of ½ lemon
salt and pepper to taste
wooden skewers
fresh herbs for garnishing

1. Cut the chicken into 2–3cm cubes.
2. Combine all the other ingredients and season with salt and pepper.
3. Add the chicken cubes and mix, making sure that they're well coated.
4. Marinate in the fridge for at least 2 hours.
5. Once marinated, thread the chicken cubes onto skewers, about 4 cubes per skewer.
6. Cook on a braai over medium coals, turning occasionally. Alternatively, heat a griddle pan, add a dash of oil and fry the chicken skewers, turning once or twice, until cooked. Don't overcook the chicken otherwise the meat will be dry. Garnish with fresh herbs.
7. Best served with *Cacik* (see page 67), and a salad of Roasted Tomatoes, Chickpeas & Spring Onion (see page 76).

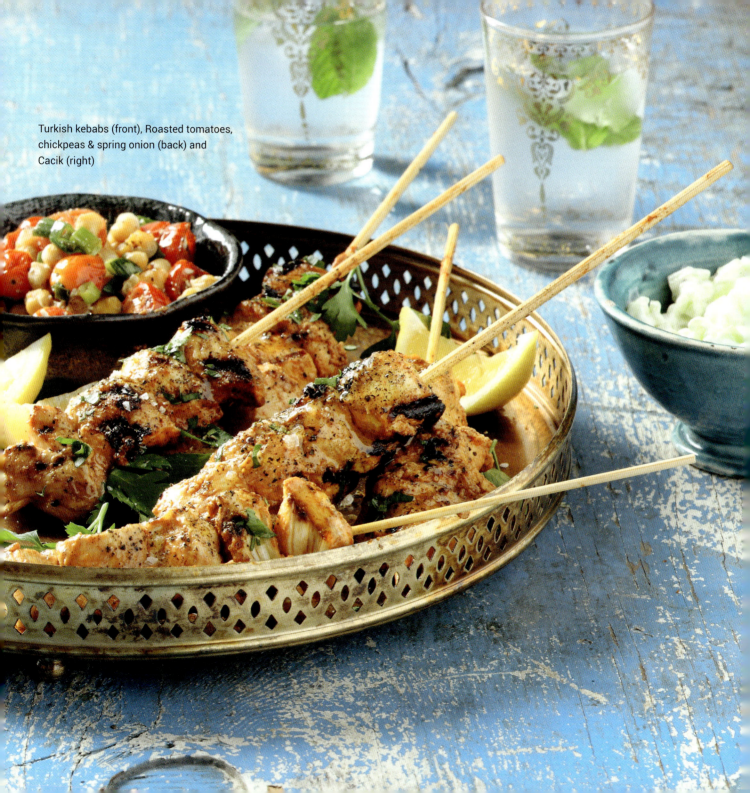

Turkish kebabs (front), Roasted tomatoes, chickpeas & spring onion (back) and Cacik (right)

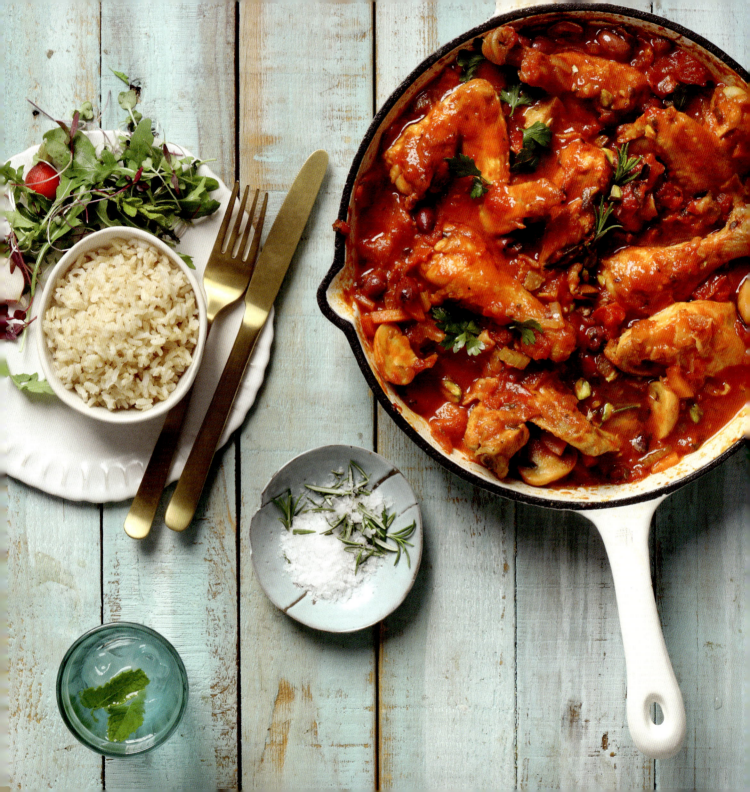

CHICKEN CACCIATORE

IN ITALIAN CUISINE, '*ALLA CACCIATORA*' REFERS TO A MEAL THAT'S PREPARED IN 'HUNTER'S STYLE' AND TYPICALLY INDICATES A STEW MADE WITH ONIONS, HERBS, TOMATOES AND WINE. HERE, I'VE USED CHICKEN, BUT IT'S FREQUENTLY PREPARED WITH RABBIT, WHICH THE HUNTERS WOULD SHOOT IN WINTER. THIS IS THE PERFECT DISH TO SERVE TO A CROWD AS YOU SIMPLY DOUBLE UP THE INGREDIENTS. IT COULDN'T BE EASIER TO PREPARE AS ALL THE INGREDIENTS GO INTO ONE POT. ITALIAN COMFORT FOOD AT ITS BEST!

olive oil for frying

6–8 chicken pieces

1 x 200g packet bacon, roughly chopped

1 onion, sliced

2 carrots, chopped

2 stalks celery, sliced

2½ cups roughly chopped mushrooms

½ tsp crushed garlic

1 cup white wine

1 x 400g can chopped tomatoes

4 tablespoons tomato paste

½ cup chicken stock

4–6 sprigs of fresh rosemary

2 Tbsp roughly chopped fresh sage

1 cup pitted black olives, halved

salt and pepper to taste

1. Pour a touch of olive oil into a casserole dish and brown the chicken pieces on the hob. Remove the chicken and set aside.
2. Add the bacon to the casserole and cook for about 3 minutes.
3. Add the onion, carrots and celery and cook for another 5 minutes.
4. Stir in the mushrooms, garlic and wine. Simmer for a further 5 minutes.
5. Return the chicken pieces to the dish, along with the canned tomatoes, tomato paste, chicken stock, rosemary, sage and olives. Stir, cover and leave to simmer for about 15 minutes.
6. Remove the lid, season with salt and pepper, stir again and allow to simmer for 25 minutes more, stirring occasionally.
7. Serve with brown rice.

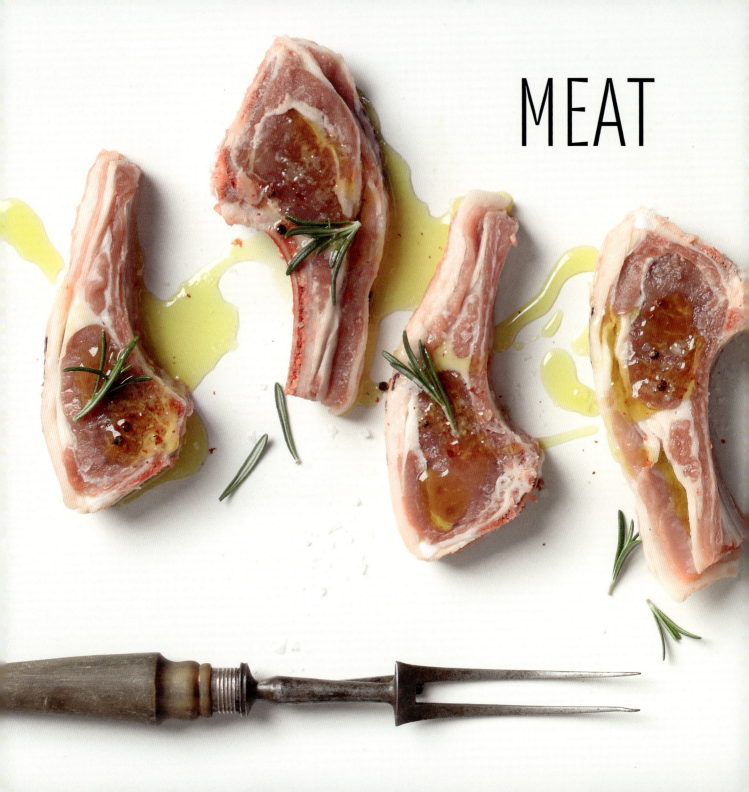

MEAT

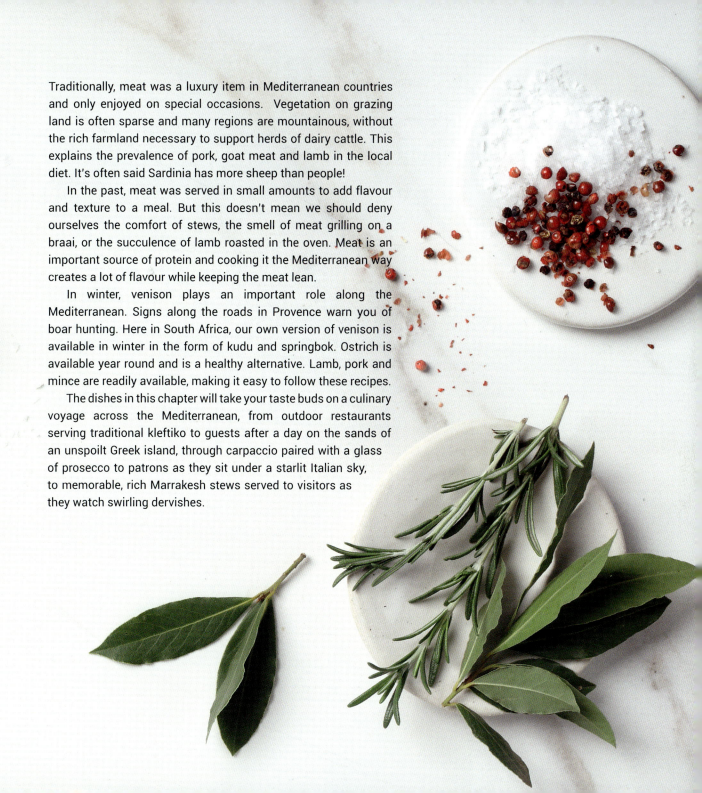

Traditionally, meat was a luxury item in Mediterranean countries and only enjoyed on special occasions. Vegetation on grazing land is often sparse and many regions are mountainous, without the rich farmland necessary to support herds of dairy cattle. This explains the prevalence of pork, goat meat and lamb in the local diet. It's often said Sardinia has more sheep than people!

In the past, meat was served in small amounts to add flavour and texture to a meal. But this doesn't mean we should deny ourselves the comfort of stews, the smell of meat grilling on a braai, or the succulence of lamb roasted in the oven. Meat is an important source of protein and cooking it the Mediterranean way creates a lot of flavour while keeping the meat lean.

In winter, venison plays an important role along the Mediterranean. Signs along the roads in Provence warn you of boar hunting. Here in South Africa, our own version of venison is available in winter in the form of kudu and springbok. Ostrich is available year round and is a healthy alternative. Lamb, pork and mince are readily available, making it easy to follow these recipes.

The dishes in this chapter will take your taste buds on a culinary voyage across the Mediterranean, from outdoor restaurants serving traditional kleftiko to guests after a day on the sands of an unspoilt Greek island, through carpaccio paired with a glass of prosecco to patrons as they sit under a starlit Italian sky, to memorable, rich Marrakesh stews served to visitors as they watch swirling dervishes.

IZMIR *KÖFTES*

THIS DISH CONJURES UP ROMANTIC IMAGES OF TURKEY, A LAND WHERE MEATBALLS ARE MADE WITH EITHER MINCED LAMB OR A COMBINATION OF LAMB AND BEEF. THE END RESULT IS KNOWN AS '*KÖFTE*' (ALSO SPELT 'KOFTA'). *KÖFTES* COME IN MANY SHAPES AND SIZES AND ARE COOKED IN DIFFERENT WAYS. IN THIS RECIPE I'VE FOLLOWED THE IZMIR KÖFTE STYLE, A TOWN RENOWNED FOR ITS MEATBALLS, WHICH CALLS FOR THEM TO BE FRIED FIRST AND THEN COOKED IN A TOMATO SAUCE. THEY ARE TRADITIONALLY SERVED WITH *CACIK*, WHICH IS A CUCUMBER AND YOGHURT DIP. HERE, IT WORKS JUST AS WELL WITH PLAIN YOGHURT.

KÖFTES

3 slices brown bread, crusts
  removed
¼ cup water
1 egg
salt and pepper to taste
500g minced beef or lamb
2 cloves garlic, crushed

1 Tbsp ground cumin
1–2 rounds feta, cut into 1cm cubes
cake flour for coating
olive oil for frying
medium fat yoghurt for serving

SAUCE

olive oil for frying
1 tsp cumin seeds
1 x 400g can chopped tomatoes
16 pitted green olives
½ cup water
1 Tbsp tomato purée
1 Tbsp dried origanum

1. Soak the bread in the water for about 5 minutes.
2. Lightly beat the egg in a large bowl.
3. Squeeze the water out of the bread then add the bread to the egg and season with salt and pepper.
4. Add the meat, garlic and ground cumin and mix well. (I find it best to do this with my hands.)
5. Roll a tablespoonful of the mixture into a fat sausage-shape. Using your finger, make an indentation along the length of the 'sausage'. Fill the indentation with a cube of feta, then reshape the meat around the feta, covering it completely but retaining the slightly oblong shape of the *köfte*.
6. Once all the meat has been shaped around the feta, lightly roll each *köfte* in a little flour.
7. Heat some oil in a pan and fry the *köftes* until brown. You will probably have to do this in batches.
8. Remove and drain them on absorbent kitchen paper.
9. For the sauce, pour some oil into a saucepan and fry the cumin seeds gently for a few seconds to release the aroma.
10. Stir in the tomatoes, olives, water and tomato purée.
11. Add the *köftes* and leave to simmer for about 5 minutes, ensuring that they are well covered.
12. Add a dollop of yoghurt onto the *köftes* just before serving.
13. Serve with Leek & Baby Marrow Pilaf (see page 69).

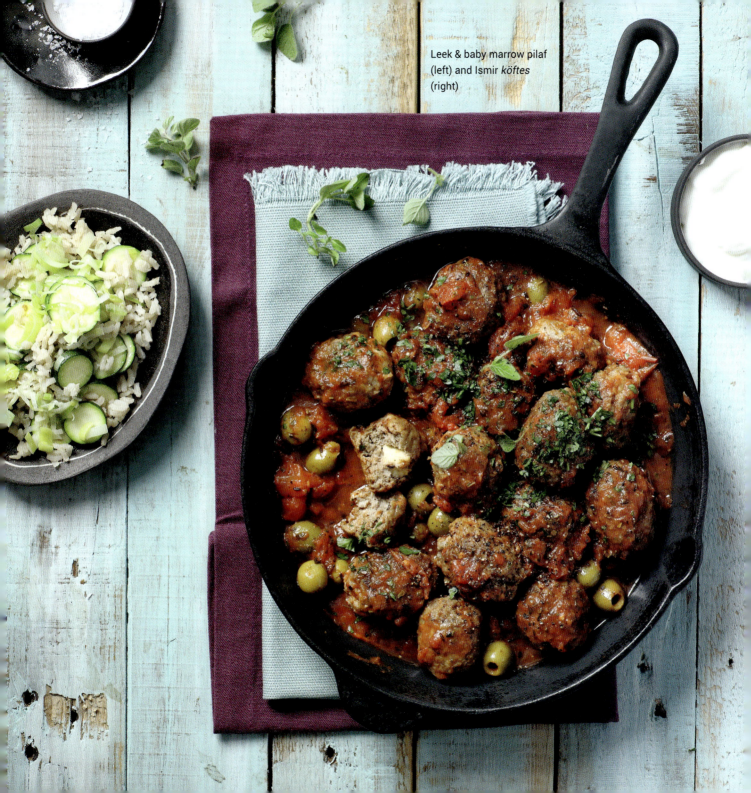

Leek & baby marrow pilaf
(left) and Ismir *köftes*
(right)

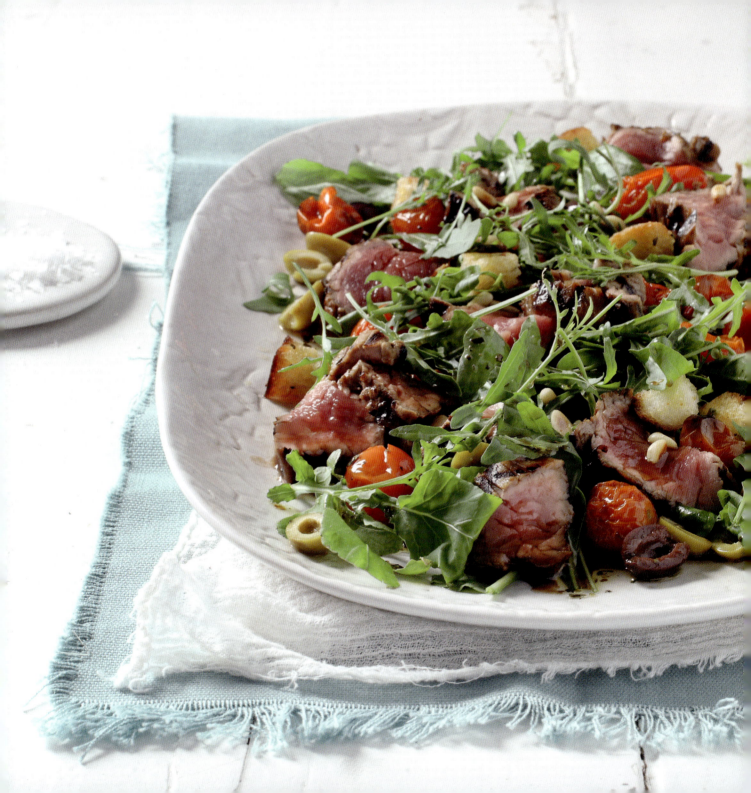

THE MED MIX SALAD

THIS DISH REPRESENTS THE ESSENCE OF ALL THAT IS MEDITERRANEAN, ALL ON ONE PLATE. THE TEMPTING COMBINATION OF TOMATO AND BASIL ALONG WITH THE CRUNCHINESS OF THE CROUTONS CONTRASTS WITH THE PLUMPNESS OF THE OLIVES, IN AN ARRAY OF COLOURS. IN THIS CASE, TEMPTATION IS HEALTHY. TOMATOES ARE A GOOD SOURCE OF LYCOPENE, AN IMPORTANT PHYTOCHEMICAL THAT GIVES THEM THEIR RED COLOURING. BY ROASTING THE TOMATOES, EVEN MORE LYCOPENE IS RELEASED, ENHANCING THEIR ANTIOXIDANT PROPERTIES.

400– 500g beef fillet
2 cups cherry tomatoes
½ cup pitted green olives, halved
½ cup pitted black olives, halved
1 cup rocket leaves
2 Tbsp chopped fresh basil, plus extra leaves for garnishing

3 Tbsp roasted pine nuts
½ cup garlic croutons

MARINADE
¼ cup sherry
2 Tbsp balsamic vinegar
2 Tbsp Worcestershire sauce
2 tsp honey
3 cloves garlic

DRESSING
¼ cup olive oil
1 Tbsp red wine vinegar
1 Tbsp honey
1 tsp dried origanum
salt and pepper to taste

1. Cut the fillet into 4 smaller steaks.
2. Combine the marinade ingredients, then marinate the steaks in it for about 10 minutes.
3. Heat a griddle pan until hot and sear the steaks on all sides. Then turn down the heat and continue to grill for a further few minutes until the steaks are done to your liking.
4. Remove and leave the steaks to rest, covered, for about 10 minutes.
5. Slice the steaks into strips and return to the marinade for another 5 minutes.
6. Preheat the oven to 180°C and roast the tomatoes on a baking tray until they start to blister. Leave to cool.
7. Combine the olives, rocket and basil leaves and add the cooled tomatoes.
8. Whisk together the dressing ingredients, pour over the salad and toss well.
9. Transfer the salad to a serving platter, arrange the steak slices on top and scatter over the pine nuts and garlic croutons.

BACON & LEEK
FRITTATA *IBRIDA*

IS IT AN OMELETTE OR IS IT A FRITTATA? WELL ACTUALLY, IT'S A HYBRID (*IBRIDA*). THE DIFFERENCE BETWEEN AN OMELETTE AND A FRITTATA IS SIMPLE. THE INGREDIENTS FOR AN OMELETTE ARE CAREFULLY PLACED INTO THE MIXED EGGS AS THEY COOK IN THE PAN. WITH A FRITTATA, THE INGREDIENTS AND THE EGGS ARE ALL MIXED TOGETHER AND THEN COOKED. HOWEVER, THIS ISN'T A TRADITIONAL FRITTATA BECAUSE IT'S BAKED AND NOT FRIED. THE FRIED VERSION TAKES A LITTLE PRACTICE TO MASTER, ESPECIALLY THE FLIPPING. THIS ONE IS MUCH EASIER AS IT'S BAKED IN THE OVEN, SO THERE'S NO RISK OF ACCIDENTALLY FLIPPING YOUR MEAL ONTO THE KITCHEN FLOOR!

---

1 x 200g packet bacon, roughly chopped

1 onion, finely chopped

3 leeks, sliced

olive oil for frying

1 cup chopped spinach

1 Tbsp chopped fresh dill

5 eggs

1 Tbsp Greek yoghurt

1 tsp tomato paste

salt and pepper to taste

1 round feta

1. Preheat the oven to 200°C. Grease an ovenproof dish.
2. Fry the bacon in a pan, until almost crispy.
3. Add the onion and cook until softened. Set aside.
4. In another clean pan gently sauté the leeks in a splash of olive oil for about 3 minutes to soften them.
5. Add the spinach and dill and mix well.
6. In a separate bowl, break the eggs and whisk them together.
7. Stir in the yoghurt and tomato paste until well mixed. Season with salt and pepper.
8. Crumble the feta into the egg mixture. Add all the other ingredients and mix well.
9. Pour into the prepared ovenproof dish and bake for about 15 minutes.
10. Switch on the grill and grill for approximately 5 minutes or until the top is golden.
11. Serve hot or at room temperature with a dollop of yoghurt and leafy greens, if you like.

CARPACCIO ON GREENS

CARPACCIO IS THE STAR OF THE SHOW HERE, BALANCING SUPERBLY WITH SIMPLE GREENS THAT ARE PARTNERED WITH THE GRAINY PARMESAN, OR PARMIGIANO-REGGIANO AS IT'S LABELLED IN ITALY. IN THIS DISH I OPT FOR MIXED LEAVES FOR THEIR COLOUR AND VARIETY. TO ADD EXTRA DEPTH TO THE FLAVOUR, THE CARPACCIO IS MARINATED IN BALSAMIC VINEGAR, ALSO NATIVE TO ITALY. THE ADDITION OF BABY POTATOES MAKES THE MEAL MORE SUBSTANTIAL; PERFECT TO SERVE TO FRIENDS AS PART OF A SUMMER LUNCH AND DELICIOUS WITH AN ICE-COLD GLASS OF WHITE WINE.

400–600g thinly sliced beef fillet
2–3 cups mixed salad leaves
2 cups spinach leaves
4–6 cooked baby potatoes in their jackets
¼ cup olive oil
¼ tsp minced chilli
salt and pepper to taste
½ cup shaved Parmesan

MARINADE
2 Tbsp balsamic vinegar
2 Tbsp olive oil
juice of 2 lemons
pepper

1. Mix together the marinade ingredients in a dish.
2. Add the fillet slices, making sure the marinade covers them well.
3. Refrigerate for about an hour, to allow the flavours to develop.
4. Scatter the salad and spinach leaves on a serving platter.
5. Slice the baby potatoes and arrange them over the leaves.
6. Combine the olive oil, chilli and salt and pepper, then pour over the leaves and potatoes.
7. Arrange the slices of fillet attractively on the platter and scatter over the Parmesan shavings.

KLEFTIKO

THIS IS GREEK CUISINE AT ITS BEST. WHO CAN RESIST THE AROMAS AND FLAVOURS OF ROASTED LAMB? KLEFTIKO LITERALLY MEANS 'STOLEN LAMB'. THE NAME ORIGINATED DURING THE 19TH CENTURY WHEN 'COMMONERS' WERE BANNED FROM OWNING THEIR OWN ANIMALS, SO PEOPLE USED TO STEAL A LAMB AND COOK IT IN A HOME-MADE OVEN; REALLY JUST A HOLE IN THE GROUND, COVERED WITH A ROCK. NO SMELLS OR SMOKE COULD ESCAPE TO BETRAY THE THIEF AND THE LAMB COULD BE SAFELY LEFT TO COOK SLOWLY FOR SEVERAL HOURS.

1.5kg leg of lamb (bone in)

slivers of garlic

8 Tbsp olive oil

cake flour for dusting

salt and pepper to taste

3–4 stalks celery, roughly chopped

3–4 small carrots, roughly chopped

1 onion, roughly chopped

3–4 sprigs of fresh rosemary

½ lemon, cut into wedges

4 Tbsp balsamic vinegar

2–3 cups red wine

1. Preheat the oven to 170°C.
2. Cut 6–7 small incisions in the lamb in various places and push the garlic into them.
3. Rub the olive oil over the surface of the lamb.
4. Dust the entire surface of the lamb with the flour and season with salt and pepper.
5. Place in a roasting pan and scatter the vegetables, rosemary and the lemon wedges around the pan.
6. Pour the balsamic vinegar over the lamb and then add about 2 cups of the red wine.
7. Cover and roast for about 2 hours, then turn the lamb and return to the oven for another 2 hours. Check once or twice to ensure that the meat isn't dry. If necessary, add the remaining wine.
8. Once cooked, remove and shred the meat. Liberally coat the shredded lamb with the cooking juices and serve.
9. Best served with Greek-style Lemon Potatoes (see page 73) and *Briam* (see page 70).

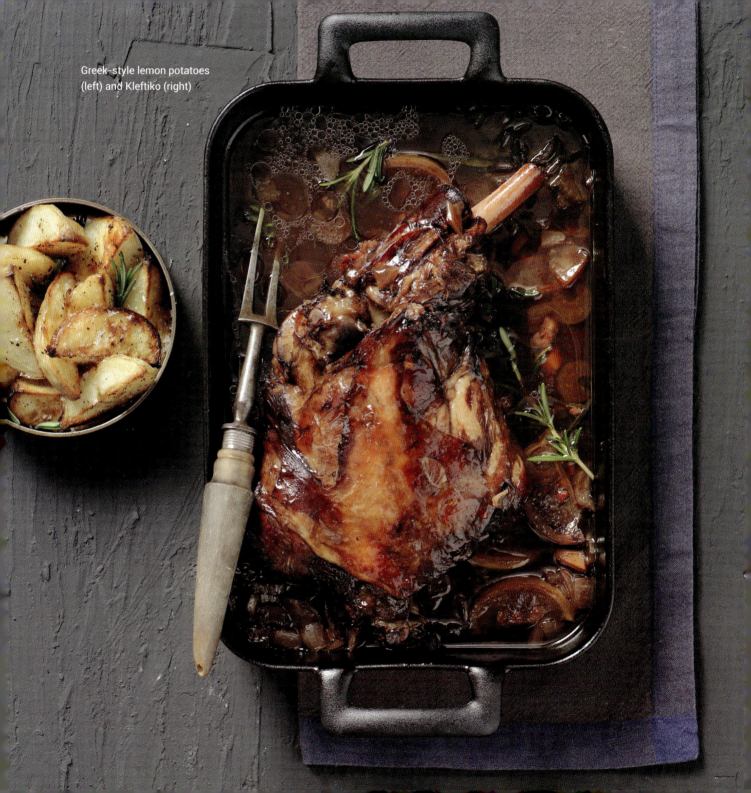

Greek-style lemon potatoes
(left) and Kleftiko (right)

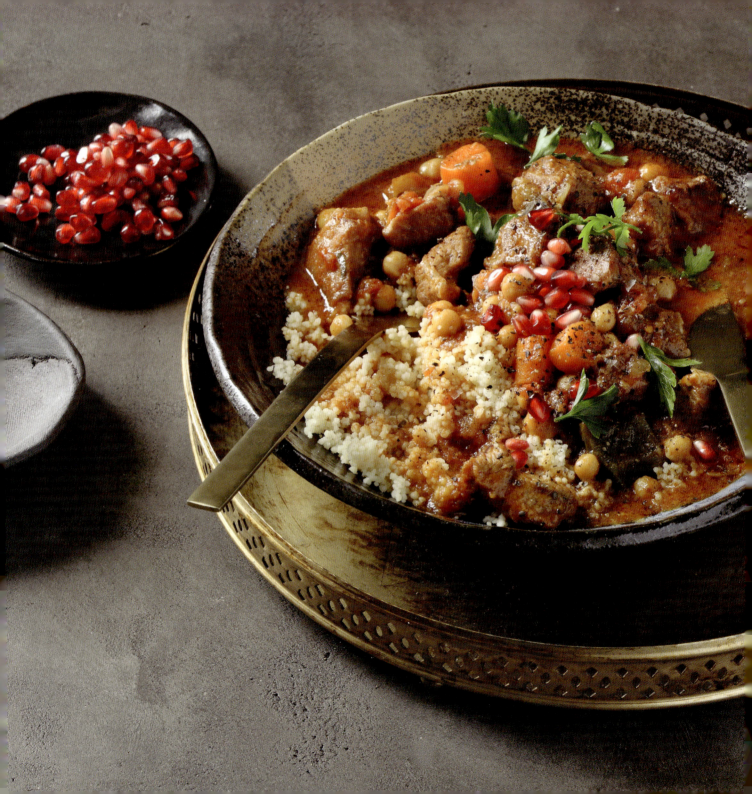

MARRAKESH BEEF STEW

POMEGRANATES, COUSCOUS, CINNAMON AND CHICKPEAS ARE QUINTESSENTIALLY MOROCCAN. HERE, THIS COMBINATION OF INGREDIENTS CREATES A DELICIOUSLY FRAGRANT MEAL THAT EVOKES THE COLOURS AND AROMAS OF THE ANCIENT SOUK FOR WHICH MARRAKESH IS FAMOUS. TRADITIONALLY, THIS DISH IS COOKED IN A TAGINE, A CONICAL EARTHENWARE POT. THE DISTINCTIVE SHAPE OF THE TAGINE ALLOWS THE FOOD TO REMAIN MOIST DURING THE COOKING PROCESS WHILE CREATING CIRCULATION WITHIN THE POT, THEREBY INFUSING THE FOOD WITH THE ASSORTED SPICES AND RELEASING THEIR FLAVOURS.

1kg boneless beef shin, cut into 1.5cm chunks and most fat removed
2 Tbsp cake flour
2 Tbsp olive oil
1 onion, roughly chopped
2½ cups chicken stock
½ x 400g can chopped tomatoes
2 Tbsp tomato paste

½ tsp ground cumin
½ tsp ground cinnamon
salt and pepper to taste
½ tsp dried mint
¼ tsp cayenne pepper
½ cup water
3 medium carrots, sliced
1 green pepper, roughly chopped
1 brinjal, unpeeled and sliced

¼ cup orange juice
1 x 410g can chickpeas
1 cup uncooked couscous
yoghurt for serving
pomegranate arils for garnishing
roughly chopped fresh parsley for garnishing

1. Dip the beef chunks in the flour and then fry them in a splash of olive oil in a heated casserole dish until browned.
2. Add the remaining oil and fry the onion together with the meat.
3. Pour in 1½ cups of the chicken stock.
4. Add the chopped tomatoes, tomato paste, cumin, cinnamon, salt, pepper, dried mint and cayenne pepper and stir.
5. Cover the casserole dish and leave to simmer for 30 minutes, stirring occasionally. If necessary, add the water.
6. Add the carrots, green pepper and brinjal and stir.
7. Cover and leave to simmer for another 30 minutes, stirring occasionally.
8. After 15 minutes, add the orange juice and chickpeas and stir.
9. Just before the meat has finished cooking, bring the remaining stock to the boil in a saucepan until reduced by half, then add the couscous.
10. Allow the couscous to absorb all the liquid, stirring occasionally. When ready, fluff up with a fork.
11. To serve, spoon some couscous (not more than one-quarter of the plate) onto each plate, ladle over some of the meat and sauce with vegetables and finally add a dollop of yoghurt on top of the meat. Scatter a few pomegranate arils on top, along with the parsley.

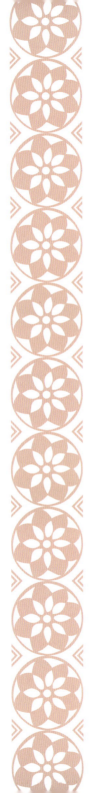

VENISON SALAD

INSPIRED BY THE RICH FLAVOURS AND BRIGHT COLOURS OF MEDITERRANEAN COOKING, THIS SALAD COMBINES THE HEARTINESS OF THE OSTRICH WITH PAWPAW, ITS SWEET PARTNER. THE SURPRISE IS THE SALTY FETA, WHICH SUPERBLY COMPLEMENTS BOTH MEAT AND LENTILS. LENTILS ARE CONSIDERED LUCKY IN SPAIN AT THE START OF THE NEW YEAR. ACCORDING TO SPANISH TRADITION, EACH ROUND LENTIL REPRESENTS A COIN, SO EATING LENTILS SUPPOSEDLY BRINGS YOU WEALTH IN THE YEAR AHEAD. VENISON IS PART OF THE CUISINE OF MANY MEDITERRANEAN COUNTRIES. HERE, I'VE TAKEN OUR EASILY AVAILABLE, HEALTHY VERSION – OSTRICH – AND PUT IT TO WORK IN THIS DELECTABLE MAIN COURSE SALAD.

400–500g ostrich steak
6 Tbsp prepared
   wholegrain mustard
¼ cup balsamic vinegar
½ cup dry white wine
2 avocados, peeled and
   cubed
1 pawpaw, cubed

2–3 rounds feta, cubed
2 x 400g cans lentils,
   drained and rinsed
4 cups baby spinach leaves
2 Tbsp chopped fresh dill

DRESSING
¼ pawpaw (leftover from
   the whole pawpaw)
¼ cup olive oil
1 tsp white wine vinegar
1 Tbsp chopped fresh basil
2 Tbsp water
salt and pepper to taste

1. Smear the ostrich steaks with the mustard.
2. Heat a griddle pan until hot, add the steaks and drizzle 1 tablespoon of balsamic vinegar onto each steak.
3. Turn the steaks over after about 4 minutes. Cook for about 3 minutes on the other side until cooked to your preference, ideally medium-rare. If the steaks start to stick to the pan, pour in the white wine to loosen them.
4. Leave the steaks to rest, covered, for 5–10 minutes before slicing thinly.
5. Combine the avocados, three-quarters of the pawpaw, the feta and lentils.
6. Add the spinach, dill and sliced ostrich. Combine gently so as not to break the avocado and pawpaw.
7. For the dressing, blend together the last quarter of the pawpaw, the oil, vinegar and basil. Add the water if the dressing is too thick. Season with salt and pepper.
8. Pour the dressing over the salad and toss gently.

STEAK *CIPOLLA*

OSTRICH STEAK IS READILY AVAILABLE IN SOUTH AFRICA SO I'VE USED IT INSTEAD OF THE MORE TRADITIONAL WILD BOAR OR ELK THAT YOU'D FIND IN THE MEDITERRANEAN COUNTRYSIDE. IT'S EXTREMELY HIGH IN PROTEIN, EASY TO DIGEST, AND LOW IN CALORIES AND CHOLESTEROL – PERFECT FOR A HEALTHY MEAL. THE CARAMELISED ONION (*CIPOLLA*) PROVIDES THE SWEETNESS – IDEAL TO SERVE WITH VENISON. IF YOU WANT TO AVOID SUGAR, USE A SUGAR SUBSTITUTE.

400–500g ostrich steaks
2–3 Tbsp prepared hot
   English mustard
a few drops of balsamic
   vinegar
¼ cup red wine

CARAMELISED ONION
3 Tbsp balsamic vinegar
2 tsp sugar
3 Tbsp olive oil
1 onion, peeled and
   sliced into half rings

1. First prepare the caramelised onion. Combine the balsamic vinegar, sugar and oil.
2. Place the onion in a saucepan, pour over the vinegar mixture and cook over a low heat for about 20 minutes, until the onion pieces are soft.
3. Smear the steaks with the mustard.
4. Heat a griddle pan and then add the ostrich steaks.
5. Drizzle some balsamic vinegar onto each steak.
6. Grill the steaks for a few minutes, then turn them over. Pour in half the wine so that the steaks don't catch on the base of the pan.
7. Grill for another few minutes and then pour in the remaining wine to loosen the steaks.
8. Remove the steaks from the pan but keep warm and leave to rest for 10 minutes before serving.
9. Slice the ostrich steaks and top with the onion. Serve with Green Pepper Cups with *Caprese* salad (see page 71).

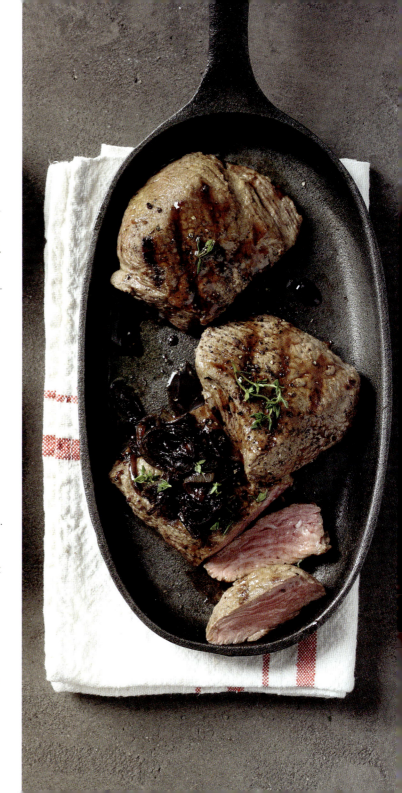

PORK *LA COL*

HAM OR PORK ON THE MENU IS A WAY OF LIFE IN SPAIN. IN TAPAS BARS AROUND THE COUNTRY, SPANIARDS DEBATE THE MERITS OF DIFFERENT BREEDS OF PIGS, WHAT THEY EAT AND THE BEST WAY OF CURING THE MEAT. APPLES PARTNER PERFECTLY WITH PORK AND HERE THEY CONTRIBUTE TO AN UNUSUAL, WARM AND DECONSTRUCTED COLESLAW. THE ADDITION OF CABBAGE (*LA COL*) AND CARROTS ASSISTS DIGESTION, WHILE THE COOKING PROCESS HELPS TO PRESERVE THE BETA-CAROTENE CONTENT OF THE CARROTS.

800g–1kg leg of pork, deboned
salt and freshly ground black pepper
   to taste
2 Tbsp chopped fresh sage
1 onion, roughly chopped
½ cup water
1 cup vegetable stock
1 x 330ml bottle cider

2 Tbsp olive oil
8 baby carrots, halved lengthways
   or 2 large carrots, julienned
1 baby green cabbage
1 lemon, quartered
1 sweet apple
2 cups baby spinach leaves

DRESSING
¼ tsp crushed garlic
½ tsp cayenne pepper
1 Tbsp Worcestershire sauce
1 Tbsp honey
1 Tbsp lemon juice
1 Tbsp olive oil

1. Preheat the oven to 190°C.
2. Season the pork with salt and pepper, then scatter over the sage.
3. Place the pork in a roasting dish, add the onion, water and vegetable stock, cover and roast for 2 hours.
4. Reduce the heat to 150°C and roast for another 3 hours. Remove the pork and leave to rest for at least 10 minutes.
5. Pull the pork apart until it is shredded.
6. Add the cider to the cooking liquid, along with the pork. Cover and return to the oven for another 30 minutes.
7. Preheat a griddle pan, add the oil and grill the carrots on both sides, until griddle lines appear, then set aside.
8. Slice the baby cabbage into quarters, but keep the base of each quarter intact.
9. Add the cabbage to the pan and grill until it starts to char. Carefully turn over and char on all sides.
10. Add the lemon quarters and cook until charred.
11. Sliced the apple into rounds and add to the pan.
12. Add additional oil if necessary and grill for another few minutes. Remove the vegetables and keep warm.
13. Combine the dressing ingredients until well mixed.
14. Arrange the spinach leaves as a base on a serving platter, add the grilled vegetables and pour over the dressing. Season with salt if necessary.
15. Serve alongside the pork.

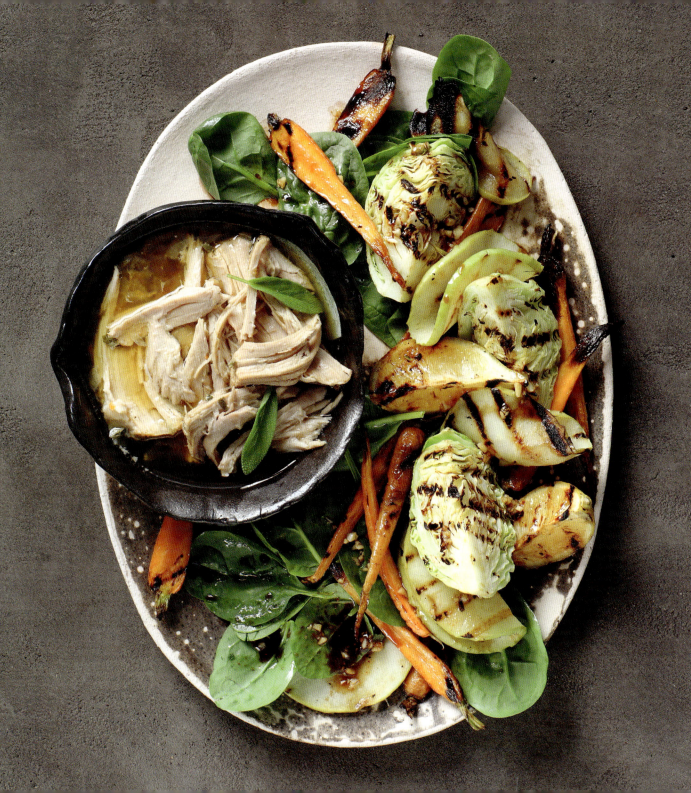

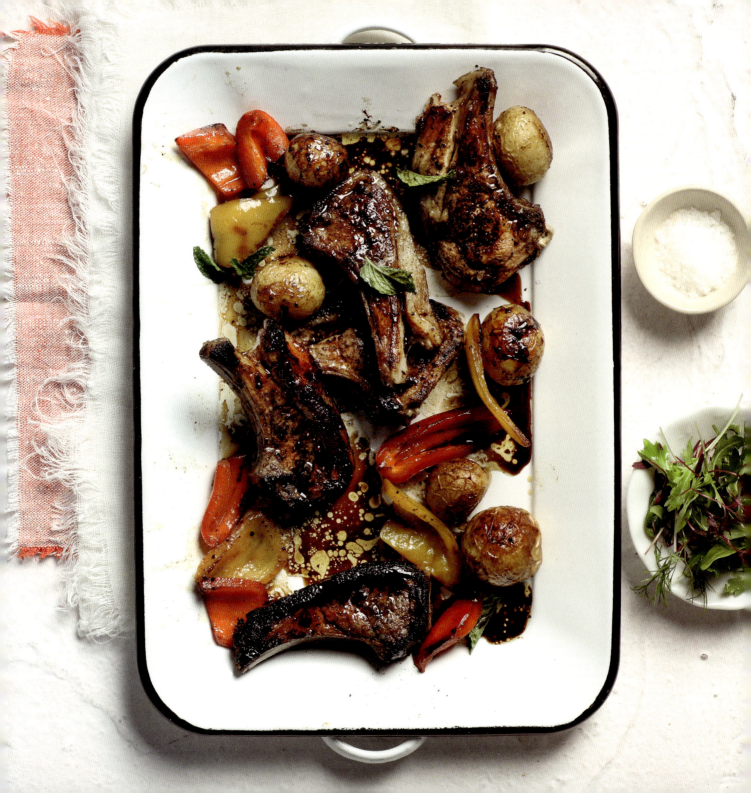

LYCABETTUS LAMB CHOPS

THESE ARE LIP-SMACKINGLY DELICIOUS. LAMB CHOPS ARE NORMALLY ASSOCIATED WITH A BRAAI, BUT THIS DISH CREATES THE CRISPINESS OF BRAAIED CHOPS WITHOUT THE HASSLE AND MESS OF AN ACTUAL BRAAI. THE STICKY-SWEETNESS OF THE LAMB, COMPLEMENTED BY THE COLOURFUL PEPPERS AND CREAMY POTATOES, IS A DELIGHT FOR THE TASTE BUDS. THE DISH ALSO PROVIDES EXTRA VITAMIN C, COURTESY OF THE PEPPERS, WHILE THE POTATOES PEP UP POTASSIUM LEVELS. MOUNT LYCABETTUS IS THE LARGE HILL OVERLOOKING ATHENS WHERE SHEEP USED TO FORAGE FREELY IN EARLIER TIMES.

6–8 large lamb chops

freshly ground black pepper

8–10 baby potatoes in their jackets

¼ cup balsamic vinegar

2 Tbsp Worcestershire sauce

3 Tbsp olive oil

1 Tbsp honey

1 red pepper, roughly chopped

1 yellow pepper, roughly chopped

salt and pepper to taste

1. Preheat the oven to 180°C.
2. Liberally season both sides of the chops with pepper.
3. Arrange the chops and potatoes in a baking dish.
4. Mix together the vinegar, Worcester sauce, olive oil and honey. Pour over the chops, ensuring that they're well coated.
5. Bake in the oven. After 30 minutes, turn the chops over and add the red and yellow peppers. Bake for another 30–45 minutes or until the fat on the chops is crispy.
6. Best served with Mangetout Salad (see page 33).

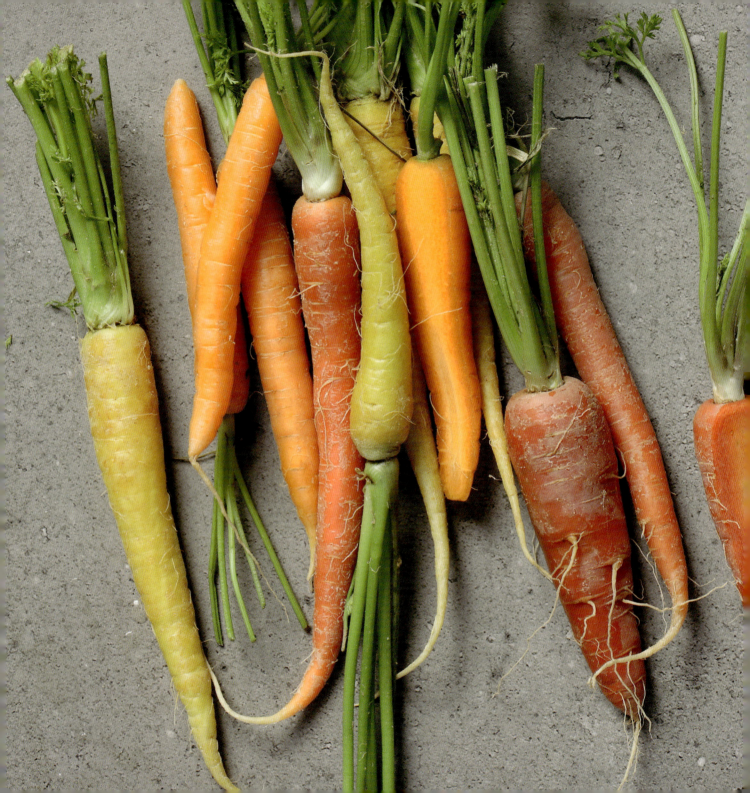

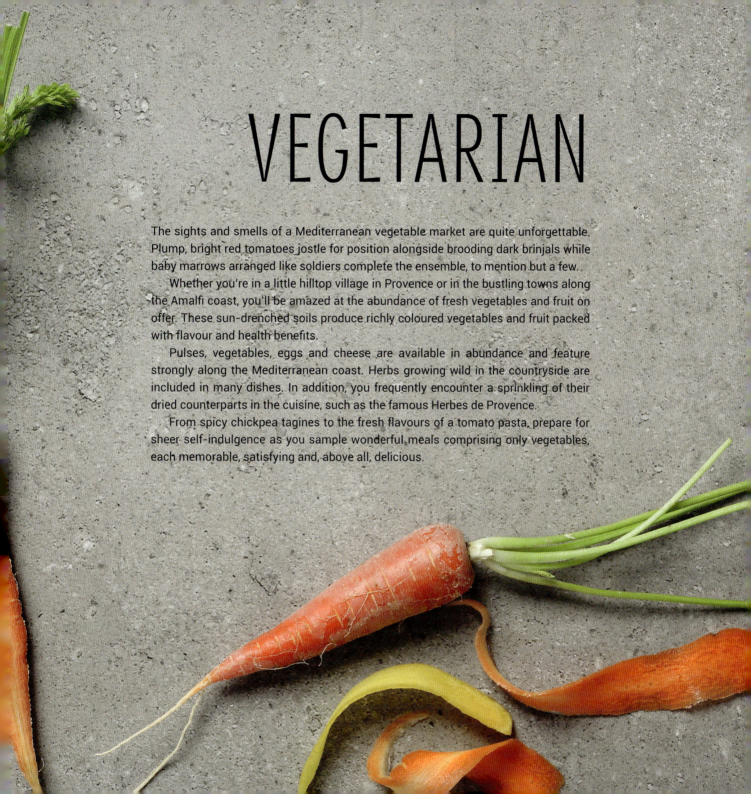

VEGETARIAN

The sights and smells of a Mediterranean vegetable market are quite unforgettable. Plump, bright red tomatoes jostle for position alongside brooding dark brinjals while baby marrows arranged like soldiers complete the ensemble, to mention but a few.

Whether you're in a little hilltop village in Provence or in the bustling towns along the Amalfi coast, you'll be amazed at the abundance of fresh vegetables and fruit on offer. These sun-drenched soils produce richly coloured vegetables and fruit packed with flavour and health benefits.

Pulses, vegetables, eggs and cheese are available in abundance and feature strongly along the Mediterranean coast. Herbs growing wild in the countryside are included in many dishes. In addition, you frequently encounter a sprinkling of their dried counterparts in the cuisine, such as the famous Herbes de Provence.

From spicy chickpea tagines to the fresh flavours of a tomato pasta, prepare for sheer self-indulgence as you sample wonderful meals comprising only vegetables, each memorable, satisfying and, above all, delicious.

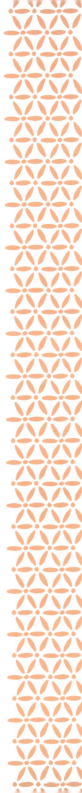

POMODORO PASTA

THIS DELICIOUS PASTA DISH IS BOTH INDULGENT AND LIGHT. THE USE OF WHOLEWHEAT PASTA GUARANTEES A HEALTHY, ENJOYABLE MEAL YET PROVIDES WHOLESOME WHOLE GRAINS. THE DIFFERENCE BETWEEN WHITE AND WHOLEWHEAT PASTA LIES IN THE PROCESSING. WHOLEWHEAT RETAINS THREE PARTS OF THE GRAIN WHILE THE PROCESSING OF THE WHITE PASTA REDUCES THE GRAIN CONTENT TO JUST ONE PART. THIS RENDERS THE REFINED PRODUCT NUTRITIONALLY INFERIOR. THE FLAVOURS OF BASIL, TOMATO (*POMODORO*) AND OLIVE COMBINE TO CREATE A SUMMERY SENSATION, WITH THE ZEST OF THE LEMON ADDING JUST THE RIGHT AMOUNT OF ZING.

12 sun-dried tomatoes
¼ cup white wine
6 cups wholewheat penne
1 Tbsp olive oil for frying
½ tsp crushed garlic
½ cup chopped rosa tomatoes
grated zest and juice of 2 lemons
½ cup pitted black olives

4 Tbsp roughly chopped fresh basil, plus
    extra leaves for garnishing
6 Tbsp olive oil
2 Tbsp white wine vinegar
½ tsp dried origanum
½ tsp prepared wholegrain mustard
½ tsp honey
salt and pepper to taste
½ cup Parmesan shavings

1. Soak the sun-dried tomatoes in the white wine for approximately 30 minutes.
2. Once softened, chop them into small pieces.
3. Cook the pasta according to the packet instructions. Drain and set aside.
4. Heat the 1 tablespoon of olive oil in a frying pan, add the garlic and rosa tomatoes and gently fry until the tomatoes have softened.
5. Add the chopped sun-dried tomatoes, lemon zest, olives, basil, white wine from the sun-dried tomatoes and lemon juice and leave to simmer for 5–7 minutes.
6. Stir in the cooked pasta.
7. In a separate bowl, mix together the 6 tablespoons of olive oil, white wine vinegar, origanum, mustard, honey, salt and pepper.
8. Pour over the pasta, then toss well.
9. Just before serving, scatter over the Parmesan shavings and basil leaves.

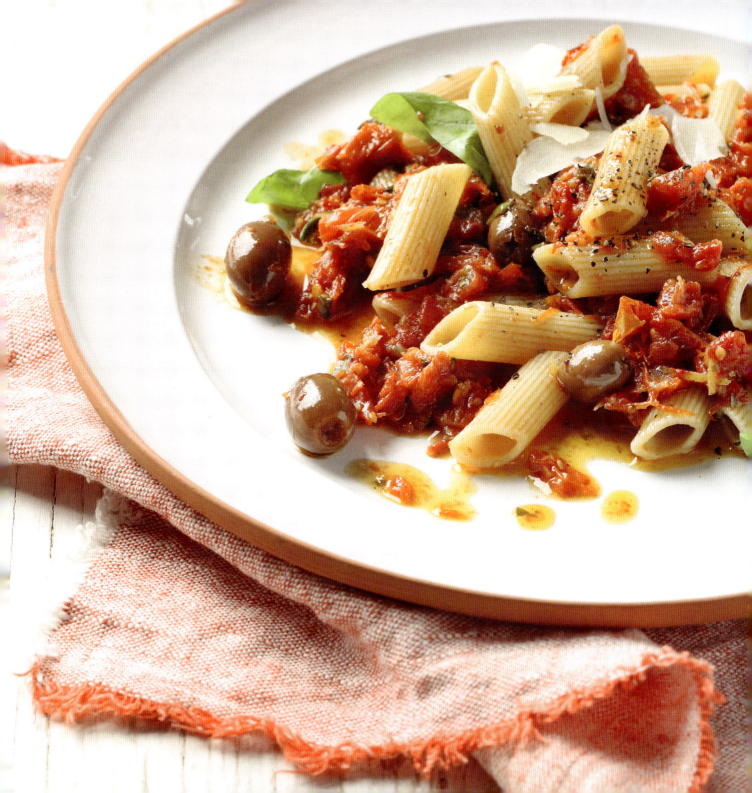

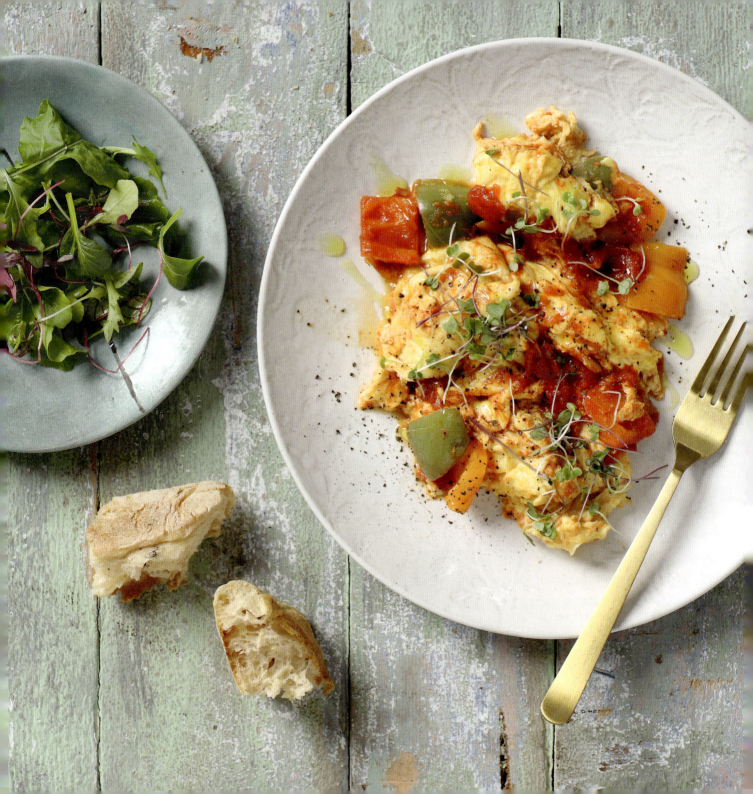

STRAPATSADA

THIS IS A POPULAR DISH THROUGHOUT GREECE, AKIN TO A TYPE OF EGG AND TOMATO FRITTATA. IT'S THE PERFECT MEAL TO QUICKLY RUSTLE UP FOR UNEXPECTED GUESTS AS YOU'RE LIKELY TO HAVE ALL THE INGREDIENTS CLOSE AT HAND. THE WORD '*STRAPATSADA*' MEANS 'EYES' – A VAGUE REFERENCE TO THE EGGS. THE HARDEST PART OF THE PROCESS (FOR NON-GREEKS) IS PRONOUNCING THE NAME OF THIS EASY-TO-PREPARE YET TASTY DISH.

8–10 eggs
¼ tsp baking powder
4 tsp Greek yoghurt
salt and pepper to taste
1 Tbsp olive oil

1 red pepper, chopped
1 green pepper, chopped
½ onion, chopped
½ cup chopped fresh tomatoes
1 Tbsp micro green or chopped fresh chives

1. In a bowl, beat the eggs, baking powder and yoghurt until well combined. Season with salt and pepper.
2. Set aside whilst preparing the pepper mixture.
3. Heat the olive oil in a pan and fry the peppers, onion and tomatoes until softened. Remove and set aside.
4. Add a touch more olive oil to the same pan, pour in the egg mixture, cover with a lid and cook over a low heat for a few minutes.
5. As it starts to set, stir in the pepper mixture and continue cooking until the egg has almost set.
6. Season to taste and scatter the micro greens or chives on top.
7. Serve immediately with leafy greens of your choice and chunky bread.

SPICY CHICKPEA & VEGETABLE TAGINE

THIS HEALTHY AND COMFORTING TAGINE IS FILLED WITH FLAVOUR AND IS DELICIOUS SERVED OVER SIMPLE COUSCOUS. YOU WON'T EVEN REALISE THERE IS NO MEAT IN THE TAGINE AS THE BRINJALS AND CHICKPEAS CREATE THE SUBSTANCE. AS IS THE CASE WITH SO MANY MOROCCAN MEALS, SPICES ARE AT THE HEART OF THE EXPERIENCE. THE UNMISTAKABLE PRESENCE OF THE SPICE IS EXPLAINED BY MOROCCO'S HISTORY AND GEOGRAPHY. THIS WAS A STOPPING-OFF POINT IN THE SPICE TRADE BETWEEN EUROPE AND THE FAR EAST. IN THE COURSE OF TIME, LOCAL PEOPLE INCORPORATED MORE AND MORE SPICE INTO THEIR OWN CUISINE, CREATING A HERITAGE TO SAVOUR.

½ Tbsp olive oil
1 onion, finely chopped
¼ tsp minced garlic
¼ tsp turmeric
½ tsp cumin seeds
½ tsp coriander seeds
¼ tsp minced chilli

1 red pepper, roughly chopped
½ brinjal, sliced and chopped into chunks
4 baby marrows, thickly sliced on the diagonal

½ x 400g can chopped tomatoes
2 Tbsp tomato purée
¾ cup water
½ x 410g can chickpeas, drained
salt and pepper to taste

1. Heat the olive oil in a saucepan, then sauté the onion and garlic for about 5 minutes or until the onion has softened.
2. Stir in the turmeric, cumin seeds, coriander seeds and chilli, then cook for about 1 minute.
3. Add the red pepper, brinjal, baby marrows, chopped tomatoes and tomato purée, then mix.
4. Pour in the water and simmer for about 20 minutes.
5. Add the chickpeas and leave to simmer again for another 5–10 minutes.
6. Season with salt and pepper.
7. Serve with couscous.

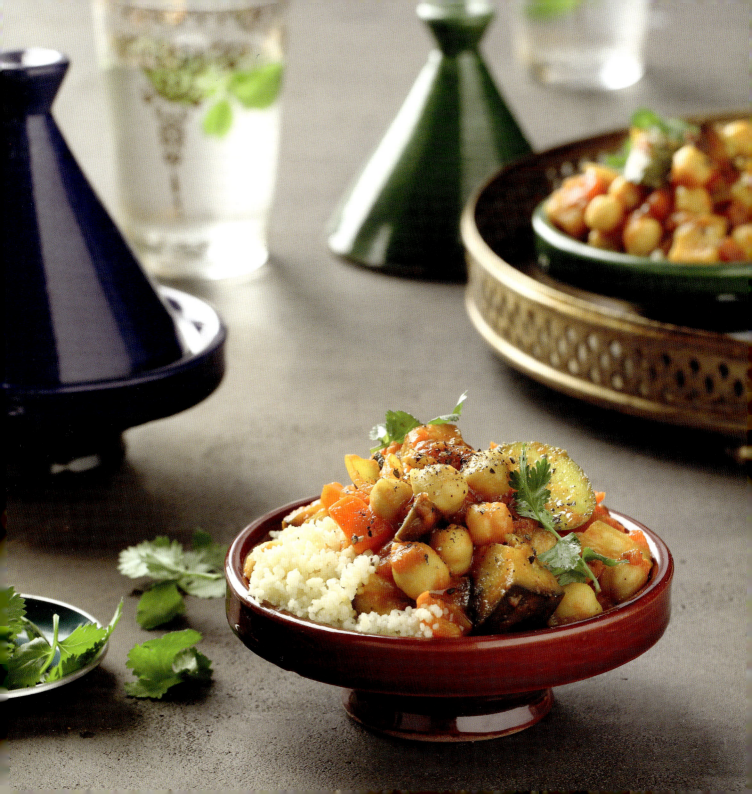

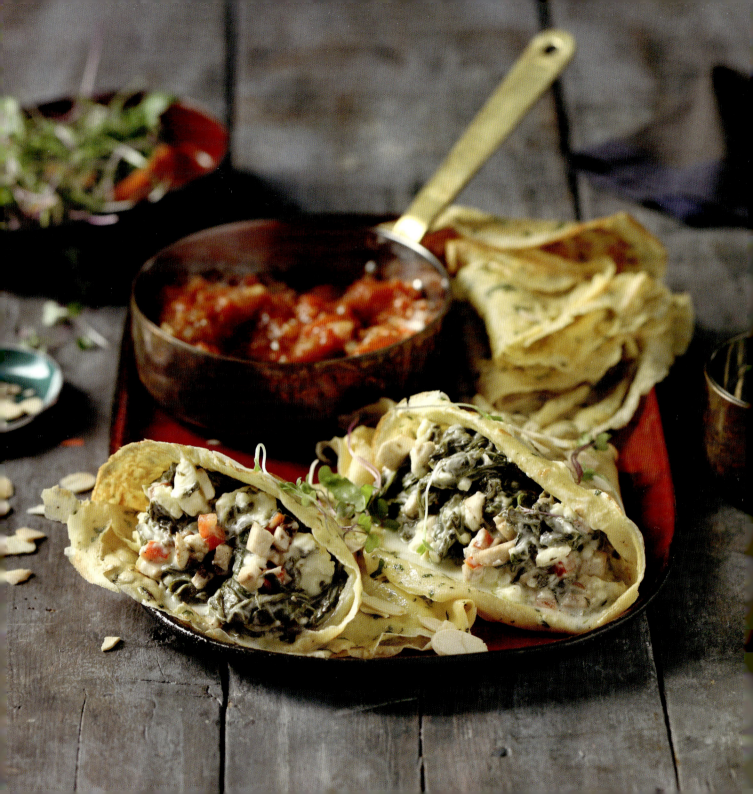

CRÊPES FERNANDE

HEALTHY MEETS TASTY IN THIS VEGETARIAN EGG SURPRISE. PART CRÊPE, PART OMELETTE, IT'S PERFECT TO SERVE TO GUESTS FOR LUNCH AS IT IS BOTH STYLISH AND FLAVOURSOME. THE USE OF READYMADE CREAMED SPINACH AND FETA ENABLES THE INGREDIENTS TO BIND TOGETHER AND ALSO GIVES YOU MORE TIME TO SPEND WITH YOUR FRIENDS AND LESS TIME HASSLING IN THE KITCHEN. NOTHING COULD BE BETTER THAN SITTING ON A SUN-DRENCHED PATIO, DRINKING CHILLED WHITE WINE WHILE SAVOURING THESE SUMMER FLAVOURS. MY HUSBAND'S MUCH-ADORED GRANDMOTHER'S NAME WAS FERNANDE; WE MAKE THIS IN HONOUR OF HER.

CRÊPES
1 Tbsp finely chopped fresh mint
1 Tbsp finely chopped fresh basil
1 Tbsp finely chopped fresh
   origanum
⅓ cup milk
4 eggs
⅓ cup cake flour
a pinch of salt

1 Tbsp olive oil
2 Tbsp flaked almonds, roasted

SAUCE
2 Tbsp olive oil
½ onion, finely chopped
2 cloves garlic, crushed
1 x 400g can chopped tomatoes
1 Tbsp balsamic vinegar

FILLING
500g frozen spinach and feta mix,
   defrosted
½ cup finely chopped mushrooms
¼ red pepper, finely chopped
a pinch of nutmeg
salt and pepper to taste

1. Preheat the oven to 190°C.
2. For the crêpes, mix together the fresh herbs, milk, eggs, flour and salt.
3. To prepare the sauce, heat the oil in a small pan, add the onion and garlic and cook gently for 5 minutes. Stir in the tomatoes and balsamic vinegar and cook until thickened.
4. To make the filling, heat the spinach and feta mix with the mushrooms and red pepper.
5. Season with nutmeg, salt and pepper and mix well.
6. To cook the crêpes, heat a large non-stick frying pan, add a small amount of olive oil and pour in a ladleful of the batter. Swirl around until the batter covers the base of the pan evenly. Cook for 2 minutes, turn and cook for a further 1–2 minutes. Make 3 more crêpes in the same way.
7. Place 1 crêpe at a time on a lightly oiled baking sheet, add a spoonful of the filling and fold 2 sides of the crêpe over, covering the filling. Bake in the oven for about 10 minutes.
8. Meanwhile, reheat the sauce gently, stirring occasionally.
9. Pour the sauce over the crêpes and scatter the roasted almonds on top.
10. Serve with fresh bread and leafy greens.

RISOTTO *DI VERDURE*

RISOTTO, FOR ME, IS QUINTESSENTIALLY ITALIAN AND IN ESSENCE IS A WARM, HEARTY RICE DISH FLAVOURED WITH STOCK AND PARMESAN. IT'S EASY TO MAKE AND SO VERSATILE AS ANY NUMBER OF INGREDIENTS MAY BE ADDED. TO CELEBRATE SUMMER, ADD ALL THAT IS FRESH AND COLOURFUL TO CREATE A RISOTTO THAT IS BOTH CREAMY AND FULL OF GOODNESS. FRESH SEASONAL PRODUCE MAKES THIS VEGETABLE RISOTTO SHINE.

½ cup chopped onion

1 Tbsp olive oil

1½–2 cups uncooked Arborio rice

¼ tsp minced garlic

2¾ cups chicken stock

½ cup white wine

½ cup sliced carrots

½ cup chopped and ribboned baby marrows or asparagus spears

2 artichoke bottoms, chopped

1 tsp dried thyme

1 tsp dried origanum

½ cup sliced mangetout

½ cup grated Parmesan

1. Gently fry the onion in the olive oil until softened.
2. Add the rice and garlic and stir to coat the rice in the oil. Fry for another 2 minutes.
3. Add half a cup of the stock and stir until the rice absorbs the liquid.
4. Add the wine and stir until it is absorbed.
5. Add the carrots, baby marrows or asparagus, artichokes, thyme and origanum, then ladle the stock in gradually, stirring to allow the rice to absorb the liquid.
6. When there is half a cup of stock left, stir in the mangetout.
7. Once the rice has softened and all the liquid has been absorbed, stir in the Parmesan and mix through.
8. Serve immediately.

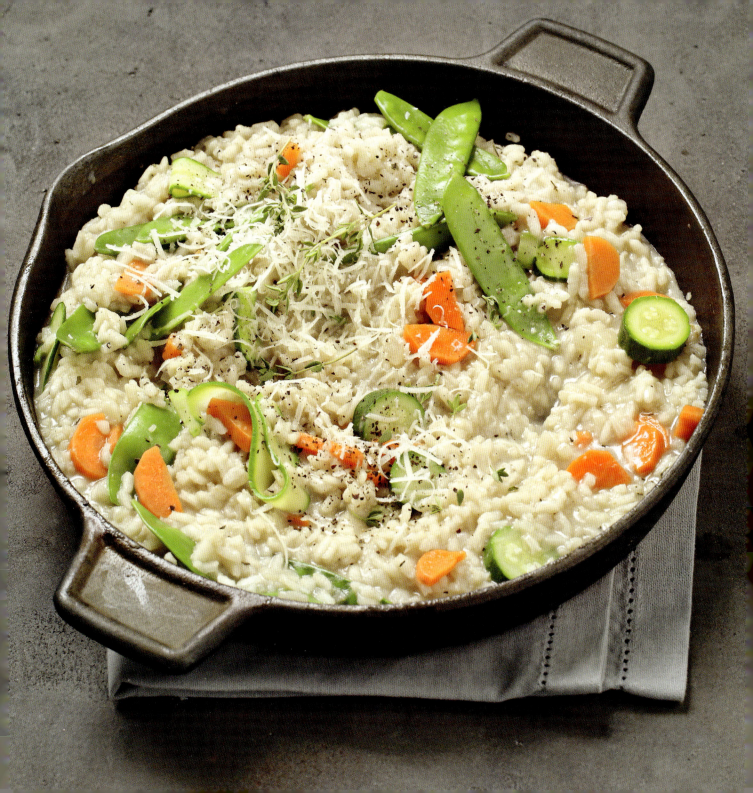

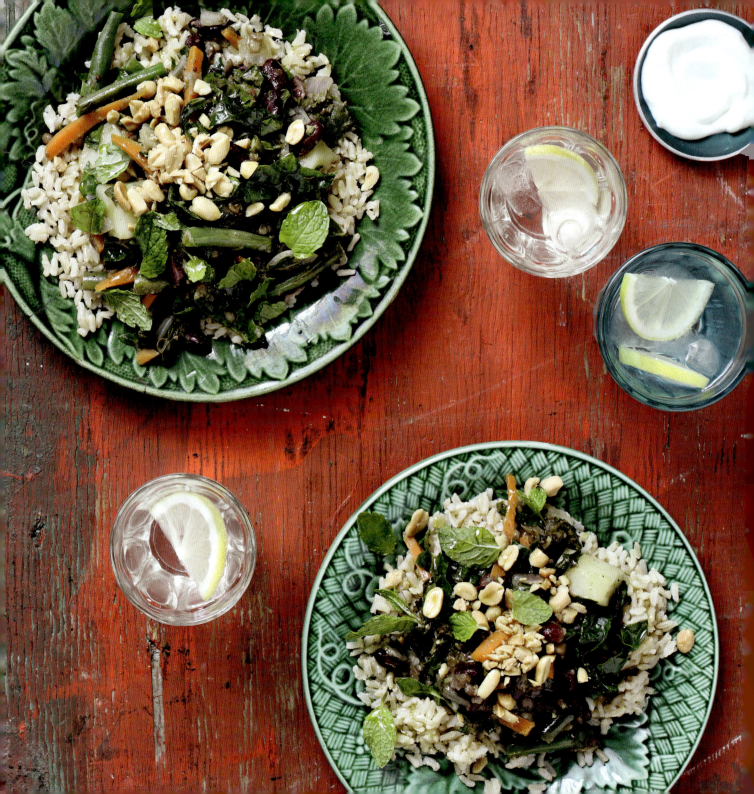

ESTOFADA DE VEGETALES

HEALTHY FOOD MEETS HEALTHY WALLET. THIS SPANISH-STYLE VEGETABLE AND LENTIL STEW (*ESTOFADA*) IS A SUPER SATIATING DISH THAT IS HEAVY ON FLAVOUR, BUT LIGHT ON COST. AS A BONUS, IT PROVIDES A GOODLY DOSE OF YOUR DAILY VEGETABLES. LENTILS ARE WONDERFULLY NUTRITIOUS, LOW IN FAT AND HIGH IN PROTEIN. AS THEIR NAME SUGGESTS, KIDNEY BEANS ARE KIDNEY SHAPED. THEY ARE ESPECIALLY GOOD IN COOKED DISHES AS THEY RETAIN THEIR SHAPE, BUT ABSORB THE FLAVOURS AND SEASONINGS WHEN THE STEW IS COOKED. THE ADDITION OF DILL AND MINT CREATES A LOVELY FRESH FLAVOUR, WHILE YOGHURT ADDS CREAMINESS. SERVE ON A BED OF BROWN RICE AND YOU CAN BE SURE YOU'RE GETTING PLENTY OF FIBRE.

---

3 medium potatoes, peeled and cubed
1 red onion, chopped
4 carrots, chopped
¼ cup olive oil
1 x 410g can lentils, drained
1 x 410g can kidney beans, drained

1½ cups vegetable stock
200g fresh green beans, topped and tailed and cooked until *al dente*
3 cups shredded spinach or Swiss chard
2 Tbsp dried dill
2 Tbsp chopped fresh mint
1 Tbsp white wine vinegar

1 Tbsp honey
1 tsp prepared wholegrain mustard
salt and pepper to taste
2 Tbsp chopped peanuts
2–3 Tbsp Greek yoghurt for serving

1. Cook the potatoes in a saucepan of boiling water until soft. Remove and set aside.
2. Cook the onion and carrots in the olive oil, until softened.
3. Add the lentils, kidney beans and stock, then heat through.
4. Slice the green beans into 2cm lengths, add the potatoes and shredded spinach, dill and mint and heat until the spinach starts to wilt.
5. Add the vinegar, honey and mustard and mix.
6. Season with salt and pepper.
7. Just before serving, sprinkle the peanuts on top and serve on a bed of brown rice with a dollop of yoghurt.

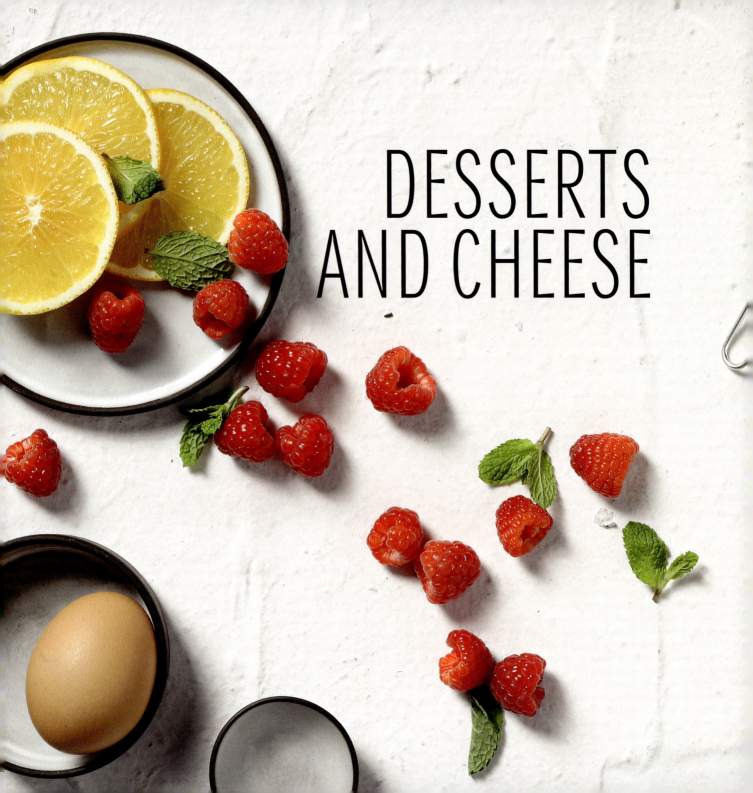

DESSERTS AND CHEESE

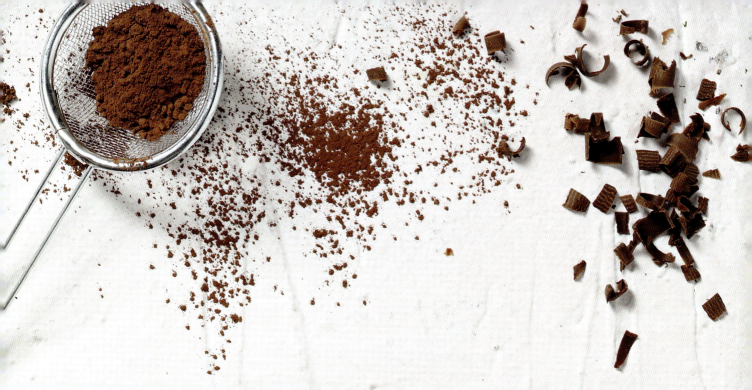

As an integral part of their daily life, people of the Mediterranean normally end their meal with fruit. So simple fruit dishes, full of flavour, make sense, especially during the warm summer months.

Whether you're in Greece or Morocco, cakes and pastries are more often enjoyed with afternoon tea or coffee. Here the Mediterranean offers a lifestyle tip with health benefits. Indulging a sweet tooth is fine, but calorie-rich confectionery items that are heavy on the digestive system are best enjoyed in the afternoon rather than at night when they will lie in the stomach during sleep.

New research has shown that chocolate high in cocoa (more than 70%) is actually good for us. It's full of antioxidants and flavonols, which are necessary to improve blood flow and lower blood pressure. But it must be consumed in moderation as it's still high in calories.

Cheese is an important element of Mediterranean cooking. Traditionally, the people along the shores of the 'Middle Sea' have eaten cheeses made from sheep's and goat's milk. But whichever cheese you prefer, it will provide a rich source of calcium, which is essential for healthy bones, and vitamin B12, which is important for the functioning of the nervous system. But, as with desserts, it must be consumed in moderation.

With the addition of crunchy nuts and sweet honey, cheeses can create the perfect ending to a meal that fits into our modern health-conscious lives.

So, whether it's a bite of something sweet and sticky or cold and refreshing, these dishes make the perfect finale to your Mediterranean feast.

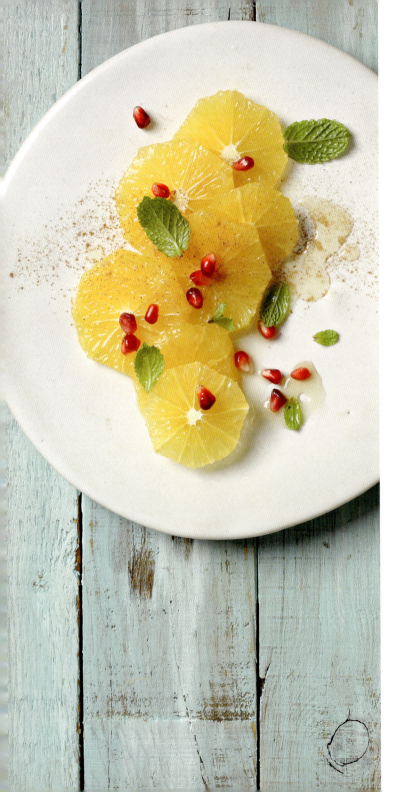

MOROCCAN ORANGES

DON'T LET THE SIMPLICITY OF THIS DISH FOOL YOU. THE COLOURS ARE A FEAST FOR THE EYES AND THE SWEETNESS OF THE ORANGES ARE HEAVEN IN THE MOUTH. THERE IS ALSO THE OPTION FOR DECADENCE BY ADDING LIQUEUR.

6–8 oranges
2 Tbsp castor sugar or sugar substitute
1 tsp ground cinnamon
1 Tbsp orange liqueur or Grand Marnier (optional)
2 Tbsp pomegranate arils
mint leaves for garnishing

1. Peel, remove the pith and slice the oranges.
2. Sprinkle over the castor sugar or sugar substitute and ground cinnamon.
3. Pour the liqueur over (if using) and place in the fridge for about 1 hour.
4. Just before serving, scatter the pomegranate arils over and garnish with the mint leaves.

FRUIT BASKETS

PHYLLO PASTRY IS OFTEN USED FOR BOTH SWEET AND
SAVOURY DISHES. I'VE USED IT HERE TO MAKE EDIBLE BASKETS,
PERFECT FOR SHOWCASING THESE MOUTHWATERING, RED
FRUITS, PACKED WITH VITAMIN C AND ADDITIONAL NUTRIENTS.

2–3 sheets phyllo pastry
2 Tbsp melted butter
1 Tbsp sugar
1 Tbsp lemon juice
1 cup strawberries, hulled, and halved if large
½ cup raspberries
2 fresh figs, quartered
whipped cream for serving
¼ cup roasted pistachio nuts
fresh mint leaves for garnishing

1. Preheat the oven to 180°C and grease a 6-cup
   muffin tray.
2. Cut out 12 squares from the phyllo pastry sheets.
3. To prepare the pastry cups, brush some melted
   butter over 1 square then place another square at
   right angles on top of it and brush with butter as
   well. Repeat with the rest of the pastry squares.
4. Line the muffin cups with the double pastry squares.
5. Bake for a few minutes until golden, then set aside.
6. Combine the sugar and lemon juice.
7. Toss the fruit in the mixture.
8. Spoon some of the fruit into the phyllo baskets,
   add a dollop of cream, scatter the nuts on top and
   garnish with a mint leaf.

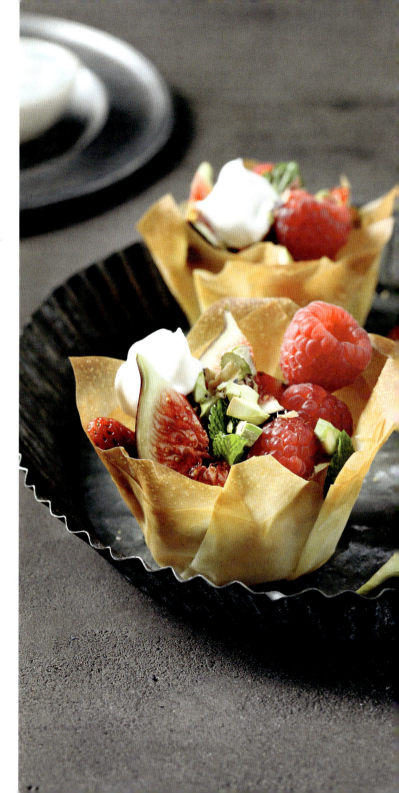

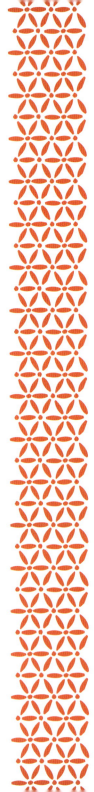

MELONS WITH PARMESAN CRUMBLE

THIS IS A COOL, FRESH DESSERT, IDEAL TO SERVE AFTER A HEARTY MEAL. IT'S PERFECT TO MAKE WHEN ENTERTAINING GUESTS AS IT CAN BE PREPARED IN ADVANCE. ALL YOU NEED TO DO IS SPRINKLE THE PARMESAN CRUMBLE OVER JUST BEFORE SERVING.

¼ watermelon
½ melon or 1 pawpaw
fresh mint leaves for garnishing
4 Tbsp dessert wine

PARMESAN CRUMBLE
1¼ cups grated Parmesan
⅓ cup cake flour
2 Tbsp butter, at room temperature

1. Preheat the oven to 170°C. Grease a baking tray.
2. First make the Parmesan crumble. In a bowl, combine the Parmesan and flour, then mix in the butter until it becomes crumbly.
3. Spread the crumble mixture on the prepared tray and bake until golden. Remove and leave to cool.
4. Using a round cookie cutter, cut out 4 slices of watermelon 5–7cm in diameter and about 2cm thick, and another 4 slices 3–4cm in diameter and about 2cm thick.
5. Using a melon baller, scoop 6 balls from the melon or pawpaw.
6. Place 1 slice of the larger piece of watermelon on each plate, then place 3 balls of melon or pawpaw on top of each watermelon slice.
7. Add a few mint leaves between the melon balls.
8. Place the smaller slice of watermelon to the side.
9. Sprinkle 1 tablespoon of the wine over the watermelon and melon balls on each plate.
10. Scatter the Parmesan crumble over the watermelon and around the plate.

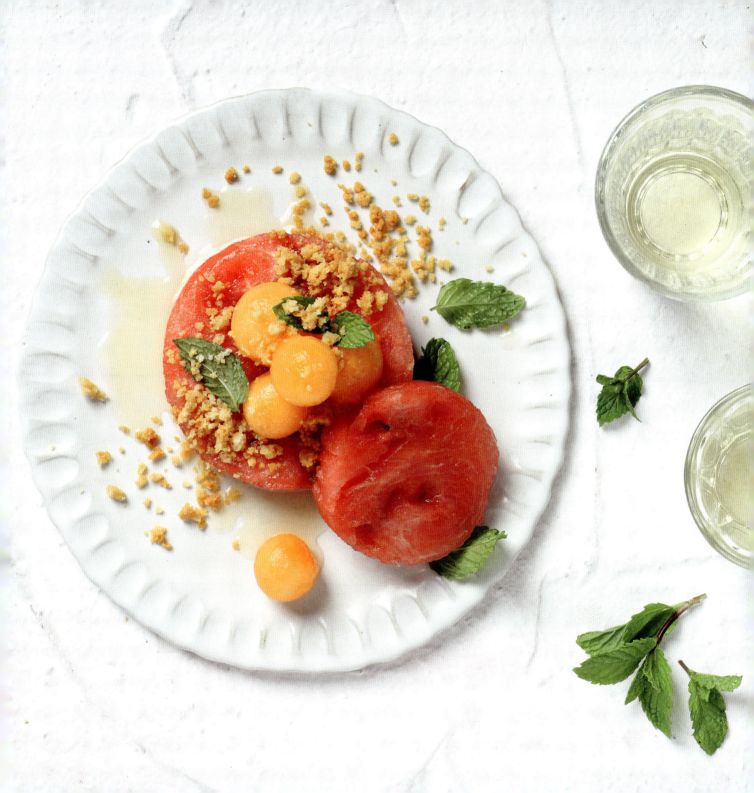

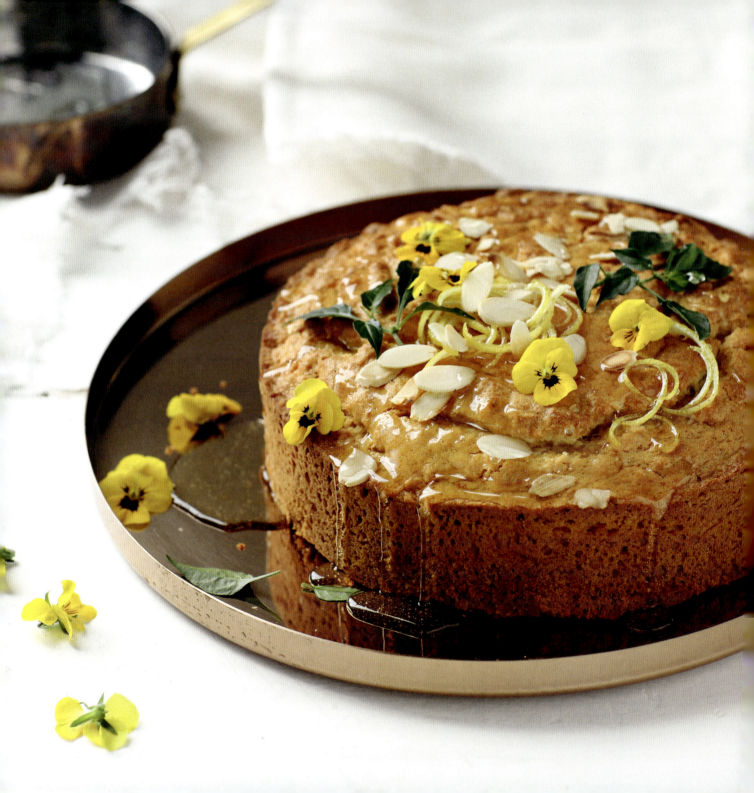

LEMON & ALMOND CAKE

TRADITIONALLY, EVERY MEDITERRANEAN HOME HAD A CAKE ON STANDBY, READY FOR UNEXPECTED GUESTS. THIS CAKE IS REALLY EASY TO MAKE AND REMARKABLY MOIST, AND BY USING LEMON AND ALMONDS I'M KEEPING IT AUTHENTIC. IT'S ALSO EASY NOWADAYS TO SUBSTITUTE WHITE SUGAR WITH THE MANY SUBSTITUTES READILY AVAILABLE IN SUPERMARKETS AND SPECIALIST HEALTH SHOPS.

½ cup castor sugar or sugar substitute

4 eggs, separated

½ cup olive oil

2 cups cake flour

1 tsp baking powder

a pinch of salt

½ cup water

¼ cup freshly squeezed lemon juice

grated zest of 1 lemon

TOPPING

juice of 1 lemon

½ cup castor sugar or sugar substitute

3–4 tsp flaked almonds

edible flowers for decorating

1. Preheat the oven to 180°C. Grease a 20cm round cake tin.
2. Using an electric mixer, combine the sugar and egg yolks.
3. Add the olive oil and mix.
4. Sift together the flour, baking powder and salt. Add to the egg and sugar mixture and beat until well mixed.
5. Stir in the lemon juice and zest.
6. In a separate bowl, beat the egg whites until stiff peaks form. Add to the egg and sugar mixture and gently mix.
7. Pour the mixture into the prepared tin and bake for 25–30 minutes or until a skewer inserted into the centre comes out clean.
8. Remove and place on a wire rack.
9. To prepare the topping, simmer the lemon juice and sugar together until the sugar dissolves. Drizzle over the top of the cake while it is still warm.
10. Scatter the almonds on top and decorate with the flowers.

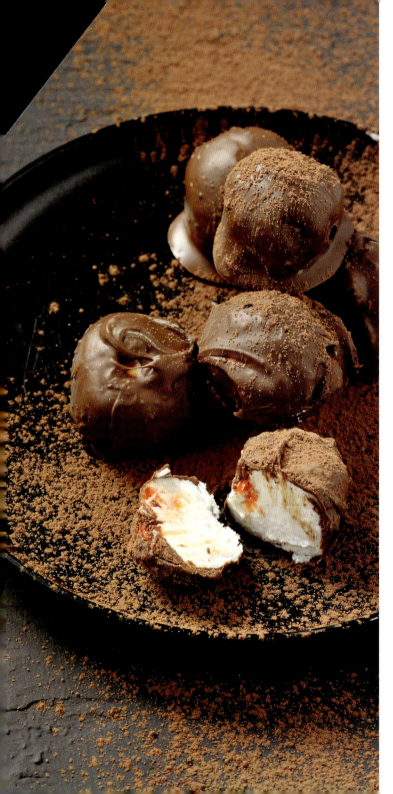

GOAT'S MILK CHEESE TRUFFLES

PART DESSERT AND PART CHEESE PLATTER, THESE LITTLE TRUFFLES WILL MAKE THE PERFECT ENDING TO ANY DINNER PARTY. SERVED ON A LARGE PLATE, GUESTS CAN EAT AS MANY OR AS FEW AS THEY LIKE, BUT I'M IN NO DOUBT, THEY'LL BE LEFT WANTING MORE.

200g goat's milk cheese, room temperature
1 tsp honey
5 hot Peppadews, quartered
200g dark chocolate

1. Soften the cheese with a fork and stir in the honey.
2. Wrap a spoonful of the mixture around a piece of Peppadew, creating a round ball.
3. Repeat until all the balls have been formed (approximately 18 balls).
4. Refrigerate for at least 1 hour, allowing the cheese to harden, which will make it easier to handle when dipped in the chocolate.
5. Melt the chocolate, either in the microwave or using a double boiler.
6. Carefully dip each ball into the melted chocolate, coating completely.
7. Remove and place on greaseproof paper to allow the chocolate to harden.
8. Store in the fridge.

HERB CHEESE BALLS

USE YOUR IMAGINATION TO CREATE DIFFERENT COATINGS AROUND THE BALL. HOW ABOUT CRUMBLED SOUR CREAM AND CHIVE RICE CRACKERS, OR TO KEEP IT IN THE SOUTH AFRICAN TRADITION, POWDERED BILTONG? WHATEVER YOU CHOOSE, IT'S A REAL SHOWSTOPPER.

100g low fat cream cheese
100g blue cheese
100g Cheddar, grated
½ onion, finely chopped
2 Tbsp finely chopped fresh parsley
2 Tbsp finely chopped fresh origanum
2 Tbsp finely chopped fresh thyme

1. Combine the 3 cheeses with the onion until well blended.
2. Mix together the finely chopped herbs.
3. Shape the cheese mixture into 1 large round ball or little balls, then roll the ball/s in the herbs until completely coated with the herbs.
4. Serve on a platter with crackers or Melba toast and some sweet chilli sauce or melon preserve.

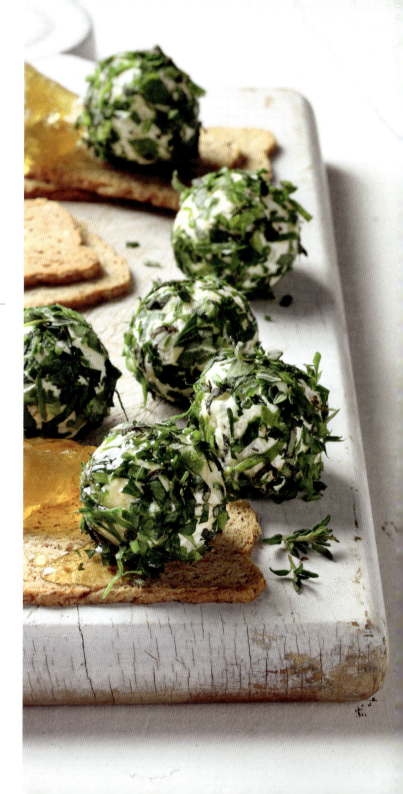

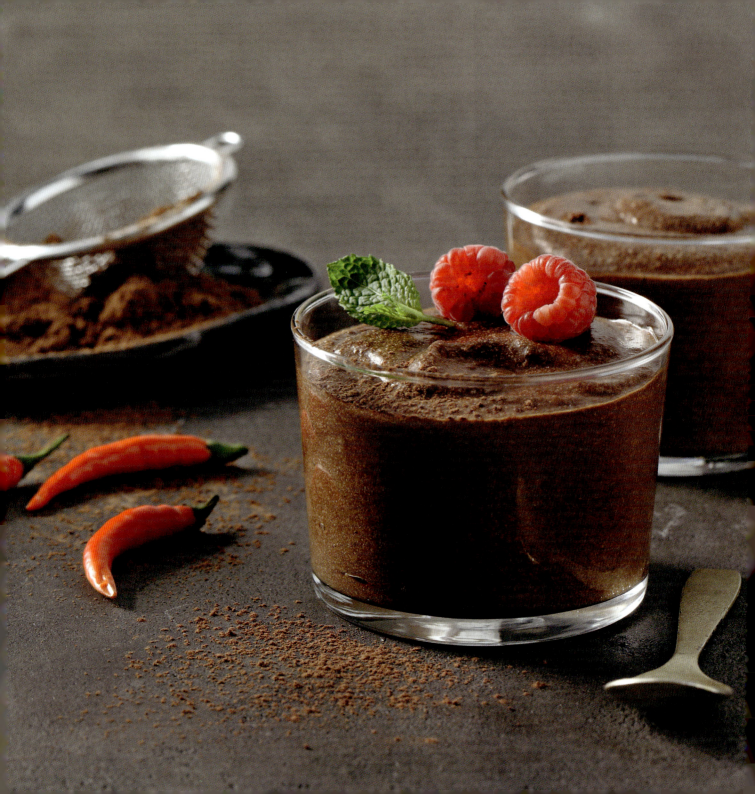

CHILLI CHOCOLATE MOUSSE

THIS IS AN INDULGENCE WITHOUT THE GUILT. IT'S LOWER IN CALORIES THAN THE USUAL CHOCOLATE MOUSSE AND THE ADDED SPICINESS OF THE DARK CHILLI CHOCOLATE IS A REAL SURPRISE. USE AT LEAST 70% COCOA CHOCOLATE TO ENJOY THE HEALTH BENEFITS.

200g chilli-flavoured dark chocolate
   (at least 70% cocoa)
2 Tbsp cocoa powder
1 tsp vanilla essence
2 Tbsp cold water

2 Tbsp boiling water
4 egg whites
½ cup Greek yoghurt
fresh berries for garnishing
fresh mint leaves for garnishing

1. Melt the chocolate in a double boiler or in the microwave in 40-second bursts.
2. Combine the cocoa, vanilla essence and cold water, then pour into the melted chocolate.
3. Add the boiling water to the chocolate and mix until silky smooth.
4. Whisk the egg whites until soft peaks form.
5. Stir the yoghurt into the chocolate mixture, then slowly fold in the egg whites. Do not over-stir or you could lose the volume.
6. Pour into individual holders and refrigerate for a couple of hours.
7. Garnish with fresh berries and mint leaves, or as desired.

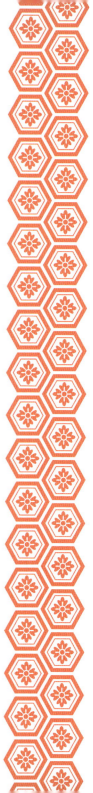

APPLE SLICES

THIS DISH IS THE PERFECT ENDING TO A RELAXED DINNER: SPECIAL YET STRESS-FREE BECAUSE IT'S SO EASY TO MAKE. SERVE IT WITH SUGAR-FREE SORBET AND IT'S SURE TO BE A WINNER.

2–3 Granny Smith apples
cake flour for rolling
1 x 200g roll readymade puff pastry
2 Tbsp fig jam
50g Emmenthaler, thinly sliced

1 egg, lightly beaten
sugar-free sorbet for serving
fresh figs for garnishing
sprigs of fresh thyme for garnishing

1. Preheat the oven to 160°C. Grease a baking tray.
2. Slice the apples about 5mm thick and place in a pot of boiling water.
3. Cook for about 3 minutes, until softened. Remove and drain on absorbent kitchen paper.
4. On a floured surface, roll out the puff pastry and cut into long strips about 5cm wide. Cut them into 10cm lengths.
5. Spoon some apple slices onto half of the strips of pastry.
6. Onto each, spread a small amount of fig jam over the apples.
7. Place a slice of cheese on top, followed by another strip of pastry.
8. Brush the top pastry layer of each stack with the egg and arrange them on the prepared baking tray.
9. Bake for about 25 minutes or until the pastry is golden and the cheese has melted.
10. Cut off any bits of cheese that might have escaped from the sides.
11. Serve about 2 slices per person with a spoonful of sorbet. Garnish with figs and thyme.

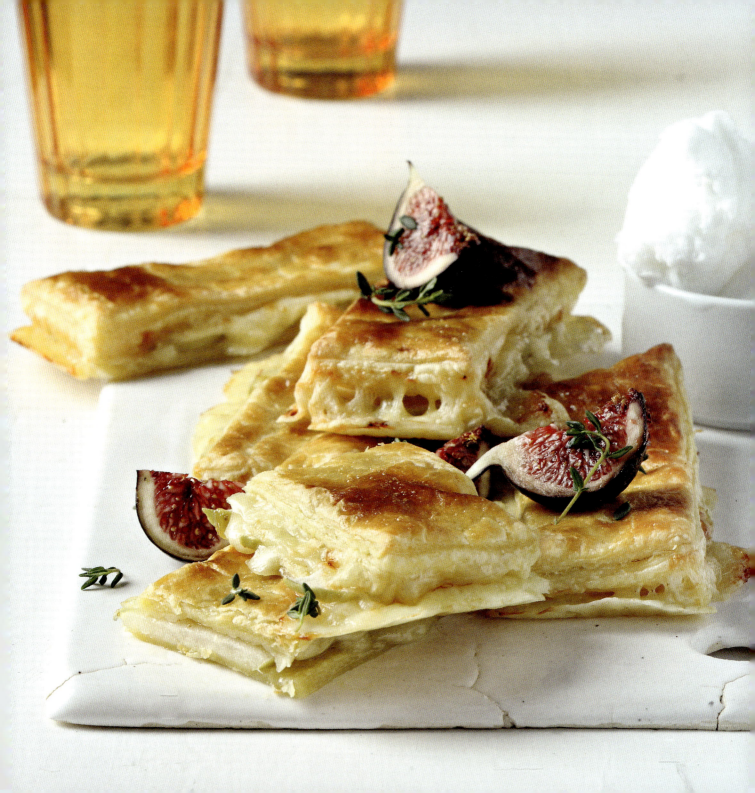

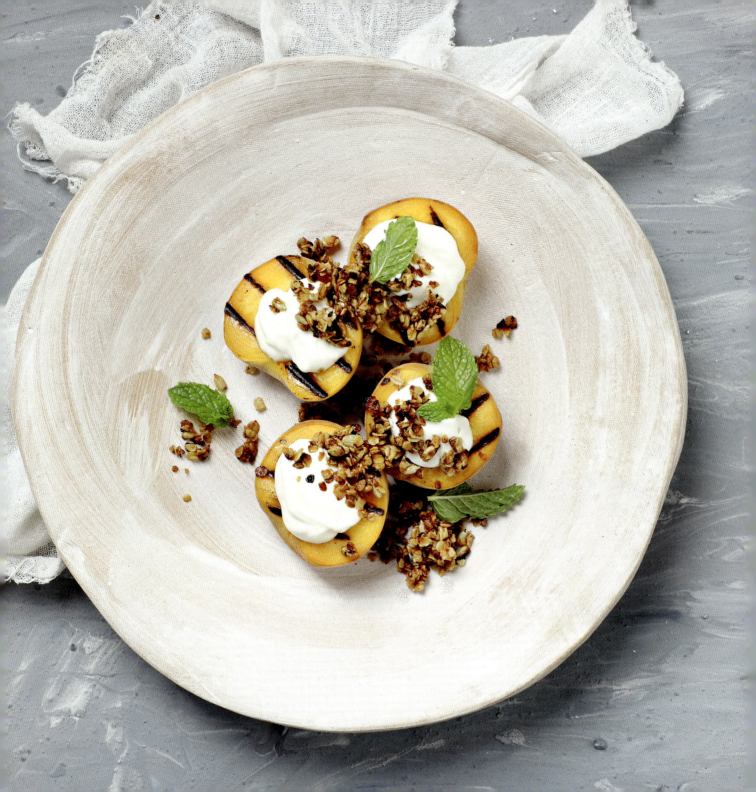

GRILLED PEACHES & CREAM CHEESE

GRILLING FRUIT BRINGS OUT THEIR NATURAL SUGAR AND INTENSIFIES THE FLAVOUR, SO USE ANY STONED FRUIT OF YOUR PREFERENCE. READYMADE GRANOLA OR MUESLI MAKES THIS A QUICK DISH TO PREPARE AND ADDS CRUNCH TO THE CREAMINESS. FOOLPROOF AND READY IN MINUTES!

2–4 ripe peaches, halved and stoned

4 Tbsp low-fat cream cheese

4 Tbsp Greek yoghurt

2 tsp honey, plus extra for drizzling

2 drops vanilla essence

6–8 Tbsp toasted granola or muesli

1. Preheat a griddle pan, place the peaches cut-side down onto the griddle and cook until just charred. Turn and repeat. Remove and keep warm.
2. Mix together the cream cheese, yoghurt, honey and essence until well combined.
3. Place 2 peach halves onto individual plates, add a dollop of the yoghurt and cheese mixture into the peach centres and scatter over the granola. If you prefer, arrange all the peaches on a serving platter.
4. Finally, drizzle a touch of honey over the tops. Garnish as desired.

CAMEMBERT CAKE

WHAT A GRAND FINALE THIS MAKES! IT MAY BE A LITTLE BIT RETRO, BUT WHO WON'T LOVE TUCKING INTO THIS GOOEY CHEESE. WITH THE ADDITION OF FRUIT, HONEY AND NUTS IT'S SURE TO BE THE STAR AT ANY DINNER TABLE. AND IF YOU REALLY WANT TO MAKE A SPLASH, TOP THE LARGE CAMEMBERT WITH A SMALLER ROUND, TO CREATE A TWO-TIER CAKE.

1 large Camembert (± 250g)
2 tsp honey, plus extra for drizzling
1 Tbsp roughly chopped hazelnuts
1 Tbsp roughly chopped walnuts

1 Tbsp roughly chopped pistachios
1–2 ripe plums, thinly sliced
2 fresh figs, quartered
1 slab peanut brittle, roughly broken up

1. Refrigerate the Camembert in order to harden it slightly.
2. Cut the cheese in half through the middle to create 2 thinner circles.
3. Spread the 2 teaspoons of honey over 1 cheese-half and scatter over the chopped nuts.
4. Place the second cheese-half on top (it doesn't matter if some of the honey drips over the sides).
5. Place some plum slices and figs on top of the cheese.
6. Scatter the pieces of the peanut brittle over the fruit and drizzle with extra honey. Garnish as desired.
7. Slice the cake into wedges and serve with a variety of crackers.

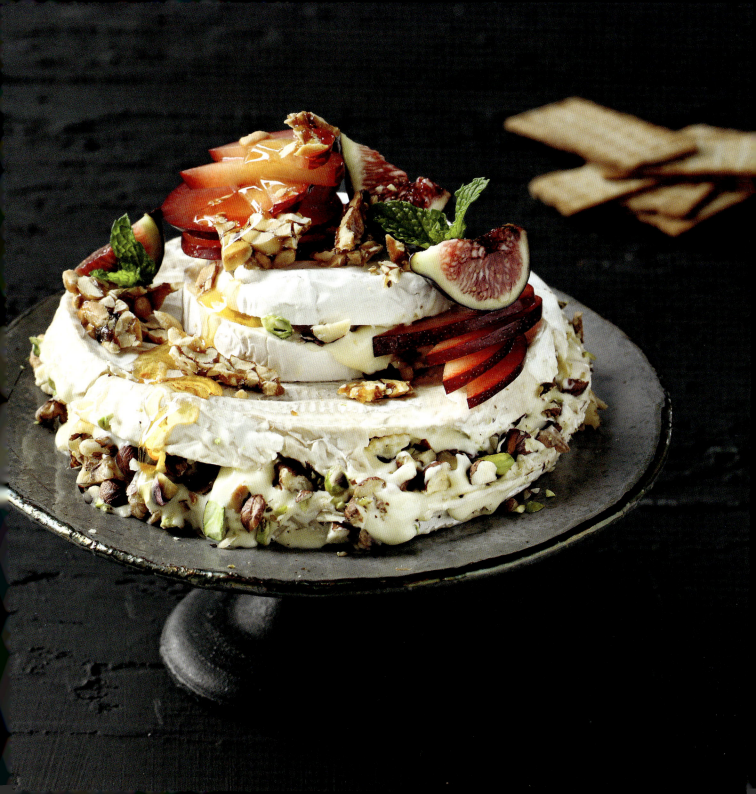

SUGGESTED MEAL PLANS

Cooking is the easy part, but deciding what to cook isn't. You've selected a main course, but you're unsure how to create a meal around it and can't decide what side dish works best or what starter pairs well.

Is it an elegant dinner to impress? Or a celebratory cocktail party? What about a bunch of family and friends to feed for lunch? Whatever the occasion, I've created these menu plans to take the fuss out of entertaining. They range from light and breezy, perfect for long, lazy summer lunches, to heartier meals better suited to the colder months.

The following are merely suggestions (not restricted to the recipes), but feel free to experiment and create your own combinations, confident in the knowledge that whatever you choose you'll be enjoying healthy, nutritious meals.

MEZE PLATTERS WINTER 1
- Brinjal dip
- Dates wrapped in proscitto
- Green pepper cups with cooked *Caprese* salad

MEZE PLATTERS WINTER 2
- Butter beans & chorizo
- Red pepper and cashew dip
- Artichoke cupcakes
- Baby marrow & ricotta tartlets

MEZE PLATTERS SUMMER 1
- *Petits pois* pâté
- Cucumber, cheese & fig morsels
- Stuffed tomatoes

MEZE PLATTERS SUMMER 2
- Oyster pâté
- Roasted chickpeas
- Brinjal with feta & pomegranates

ELEGANT LUNCH WINTER 1
- Venison salad (starter)
- Marseille seafood stew (main)
- Potato stacks (side)

ELEGANT LUNCH WINTER 2
- Chicken Véronique (main)
- Green beans with mushrooms (side)
- Thyme-flavoured baby leeks (side)
- Apple slices (dessert)

ELEGANT DINNER WINTER 1
- Artichoke & tomato towers (starter)
- Pork *la col* (main)
- Moroccan oranges (dessert)

ELEGANT DINNER WINTER 2
- Artichoke soup (starter)
- Steak *cipolla* (main)
- Parmesan mushrooms (side)
- Green pepper cups with cooked *Caprese* salad (side)

CASUAL LUNCH WINTER 1
- French onion soup (starter)
- Hake with *fystikia* crust (main)
- Broccoli, tomatoes & olives (side)

CASUAL LUNCH WINTER 2
- Fez chicken with honey (main)
- Green peppers with capers (side)
- Couscous (side)
- Apple slices (dessert)

CASUAL DINNER WINTER 1
- Valencia-style paella (main)
- Baby marrows & bacon with pesto (side)
- Red onions with capers (side)
- Chilli chocolate mousse (dessert)

CASUAL DINNER WINTER 2
- Kleftiko (main)
- *Briam* (side)
- Greek-style lemon potatoes (side)
- Moroccan oranges (dessert)

ELEGANT LUNCH SUMMER 1
- Goat's milk cheese salad (starter)
- Amalfi tomato tuna (main)
- Melons with Parmesan crumble (dessert)

ELEGANT LUNCH SUMMER 2
- Brinjal with red pepper topping (side)
- Carpaccio on greens (main)
- Grilled peaches & cream cheese (dessert)

ELEGANT DINNER SUMMER 1
- Artichoke cupcakes (starter)
- Salmon with vegetables Provençal (main)
- Risotto *di verdure* (side)
- Camembert cake (dessert)

ELEGANT DINNER SUMMER 2
- Watermelon & beetroot gazpacho (starter)
- Cannes chicken phyllo parcels (main)
- Grilled asparagus (side)
- Fruit baskets (dessert)

CASUAL LUNCH SUMMER 1
- Chilled cucumber soup (starter)
- Bacon & leek frittata *ibrida* (main)
- Spinach & raisin salad (side)

CASUAL LUNCH SUMMER 2
- Baby marrow & ricotta tartlets (starter)
- Chicken *lemnos* (main)
- Brinjal, tomato & cucumber salad (side)

CASUAL DINNER SUMMER 1
- Chicken Ramblas (main)
- Italian *piccolo* salad (side)
- Fennel *limone* (side)
- Goat's milk cheese truffles (dessert)

CASUAL DINNER SUMMER 2
- Lycabettus lamb chops (main)
- Mangetout salad (side)
- Lentil & rice salad (side)

BUFFET LUNCH WINTER 2
- Chicken cacciatore (main)
- Chermoula fish salad (main)
- Spicy chickpea & vegetable tagine (main)
- Bulgur wheat salad (side)
- Stuffed gem squash (side)

BUFFET LUNCH WINTER 2
- Marrakesh beef stew (main)
- *Estofada de vegetales* (main)
- Stuffed tomatoes (side)

BUFFET LUNCH SUMMER 1
- Pasta *pollo* (main)
- *Ensalada de Mariscos* (main)
- Cycladic tuna croquettes with baby marrows (main)
- The Med mix salad (main)
- Herb cheese balls (dessert)

BUFFET LUNCH SUMMER 2
- Izmir *köftes* (main)
- Turkish kebabs (main)
- Leek & baby marrow pilaf (side)
- *Cacik* (side)
- Roasted tomatoes, chickpeas & spring onion (side)
- Stuffed long peppers (side)
- Fruit baskets (dessert)

RECIPE INDEX

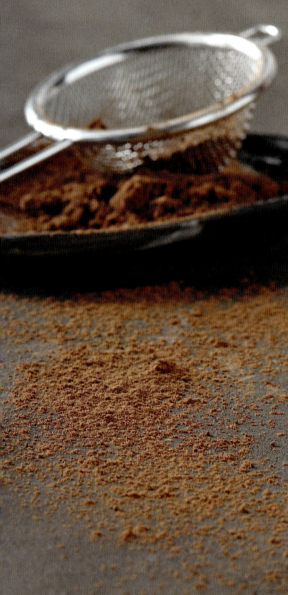